PRAISE FOR *MAKING FRIENDS WITH ANXIETY:*

'Simple, lucid advice on how to accept your anxiety.'
Matt Haig, Sunday Times Bestselling Author *of Reasons to Stay Alive*

'Sarah's advice is very sage. Deeply personal, yet eminently practical, this accessible and engaging book should prove extremely helpful to anyone trying to cope with anxiety.'
Dr Ian Williams, GP and author

'A self-help book packed with tips, exercises, and insights to ease worry and panic, this reads like chatting with an old friend; one with wit, wisdom and experience. Perfect for anyone suffering from this difficult disorder.'
The Book Doctor, Brighton and Hove Independent

PRAISE FOR *MAKING FRIENDS WITH YOUR FERTILITY*:

'An important and illuminating book, not just for those struggling with fertility, but for anyone keen to better understand the emotional impact of having – or not having – children. **Making Friends with your Fertility** is a book to read and absorb in stages and then return to. Grounded by tips and illustrations, it makes complex concepts really accessible. Simply brilliant.'
Anya Sizer, Fertility Coach, Fertility Network UK

PRAISE FOR SARAH RAYNER:

'Brilliant... Warm and approachable.' **Essentials**

'Carefully crafted and empathetic.' **Sunday Times**

'A sympathetic insight into the causes and effects of mental ill-health as it affects ordinary people. Powerful.' **My Weekly**

'Explores an emotive subject with great sensitivity.' **Sunday Express**

1

Making Friends: A series of warm, supportive guides to help you on life's journey

Sarah Rayner
Making Friends with Anxiety:
A warm, supportive little book to help ease worry and panic

Sarah Rayner
More Making Friends with Anxiety:
Discover simple ways to occupy your hands and calm your mind

Sarah Rayner, Kate Harrison and Dr Patrick Fitzgerald
Making Peace with Depression:
A warm, supportive little book to lift low mood and ease despair

Sarah Rayner and Dr Patrick Fitzgerald
Making Peace with the End of Life:
A warm, supportive guide to separating and starting anew

Sarah Rayner and Tracey Sainsbury
Making Friends with your Fertility:
A clear and comforting guide to reproductive health

Sarah Rayner and Pia Pasternack
Making Peace with Divorce:
A warm and wise companion to recovery

Sarah Rayner and Jules Miller
Making Friends with Anxiety: A Calming Colouring Book

SARAH RAYNER
with Dr Patrick Fitzgerald

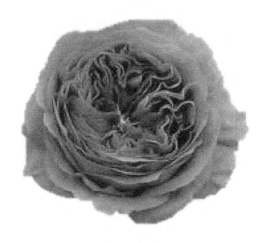

Making Friends
with the Menopause

A clear and comforting guide to support
you as your body changes

2020 edition with reference to the latest 'NICE' guidelines

First published March 2015.
2nd edition March 2016, 3rd edition March 2017, 4th edition Nov 2017,
5th edition May 2018, 6th edition Nov 2019

This edition first published in 2019 by Creative Pumpkin Publishing, an imprint of The Creative Pumpkin Ltd., 5 Howard Terrace, Brighton, East Sussex, BN1 3TR. **www.creativepumpkinpublishing.com**

Creative Pumpkin
Publishing

Cover image: Madelyn Mulvaney
Design: Sarah Rayner
All photographs by Sarah Rayner unless otherwise credited. See page 190 for a full list of sources.

www.sarah-rayner.com

Publisher's Note:

Making Friends with the Menopause provides information on a wide range of health and medical matters, but is not intended as a substitute for professional diagnosis. Any person with a condition or symptoms requiring medical attention should consult a fully qualified practitioner or therapist. While the advice and information in the book are believed to be accurate and true at the time of going to press, neither of the authors can accept any legal responsibility or liability for any errors or omissions that may have been made, nor for any inaccuracies nor for any loss, harm or injury that comes from following instructions of advice in this book.

Hello and Welcome

Night sweats, mood swings, weight gain, a reduced sex drive – these are a few effects of the menopause, although most women don't suffer them all. The purpose of this guide is to help you understand why stopping menstruating causes your body to react in a myriad of ways and to manage any particularly aggravating physical symptoms. It also aims to explore the psychological impact of the transition and ease the emotional experience, so you feel better about yourself overall. But before we attempt to navigate these sometimes murky waters, let me and my co-author introduce ourselves, so you know who's at the helm of this little book.

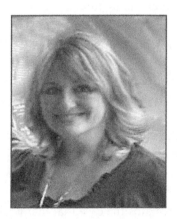

I'm **Sarah Rayner**, and my day (and sometimes night) job is as an author – some of you may know my bestselling novel *One Moment, One Morning,* or the follow-ups, *The Two Week Wait* and *Another Night, Another Day*. Alternatively, you might have come across my other non-fiction titles: *Making Friends with Anxiety* and its sister books, which include *Making Friends with your Fertility, Making Peace with Depression* and *Making Peace with Divorce*.

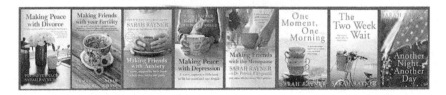

It's mainly because my anxiety became far worse in my late forties that I became interested in the menopause and its impact on our minds and bodies. Prior to this, I'll admit I could have summed up my knowledge of 'the change' on the back of a rather small envelope. But when I discovered **making friends with anxiety, rather than fighting or ignoring it, helped hugely, it set me thinking. Might such an approach ease the experience of the menopause too?** I believe it can, and this, in a nutshell, is my personal motivation for writing this book.

Yet before we go any further, another admission: I'm not a medical expert. Luckily, I know a man who is.

Patrick Fitzgerald currently works as a GP in a small town in Cheshire. We have been friends for 20 years, and feel that together our experience makes a good combination.

- **I've been through the menopause.** I'm 55 and my body is still changing.
- **Patrick has consulted patients about their menopause-related concerns on a daily basis** in his work as a GP.

Like me, Patrick believes that there is a dearth of concise, clear information available on the subject of the menopause. Although this situation was improved by the publication of clinical management and treatment guidelines by the UK National Institute of Health and Care Excellence (NICE), it remains the case that many women feel uncertain and worried about the effects of change.

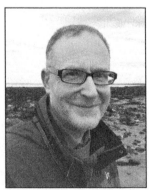

Photograph by Karl Harris

Patrick and I don't agree on everything (cats v. dogs, for instance), nonetheless we feel this book is important because:

1. **Ignoring the menopause won't make it go away**. Instead, understanding the changes you're going through will make the process less daunting and scary.

2. **The menopause is not 'the end' of womanhood, or of sexual activity and attractiveness**. It's part of our life journey as women. In many ways it's a cause for celebration, as with age come wisdom and insight. But…

3. **We know some ways that may make the journey easier** and would like to pass them on. No matter if you're just beginning to notice your body changing or are right in the middle of the process and suffering a great deal, *Making Friends with the Menopause* aims to help you work out the best way through.

4. **We aim to reflect the most salient points from the NICE guidelines** in this 2020 edition. You'll find Patrick's summary on page 29-30.

5. **We won't make false promises.** *Making Friends with the Menopause* isn't going to *cure* all your symptoms. The menopause is a natural process and we can no sooner make it go away completely than give you the elixir of everlasting life.

6. **I aim to ask some of the trickier questions you might like to ask a doctor yourself, and Patrick aims to answer as best he can**. You'll find our Q&A in grey panels.

7. **No two people are alike**, so we invited many women, each of whom was at a different stage of the process, to share how the menopause has affected them, and their experiences are included.

8. **There's also a *Making Friends with the Menopause* Facebook group**. This isn't mediated by a doctor (Patrick has a surgery to run), but it IS a place to share experiences, insights and ask questions of other women in confidence. Since this book was published, the group has grown hugely. We've nearly 3000 very active members and we hope you will find it a source of support. Find it at https://www.facebook.com/groups/makingfriends withthemenopause/

9. **This guide is divided into nine chapters**. Together they make up the word 'M.E.N.O.P.A.U.S.E.', starting with 'M' for Menstruation and finishing with 'E' for Emergence. This approach is designed to reflect the journey women go through and make it easier to absorb the contents of the book.

10. ***Making Friends with the Menopause* is relatively concise**. Think of it as a GCSE or 'O' level in the menopause – by the time you've finished, you'll have a good overview. Afterwards, if you want to explore the subject in more detail, we'd encourage that.

11. **You can dip into this guide as and when you need to**. Whilst we'd love you to read it from start to finish and digest every word, we appreciate some chapters are bound to be more relevant to you than others, so please feel free to focus on specific sections and skim passages accordingly.

12. **There is also a list of websites and further recommended reading at the end**, and in the digital version you will find direct links to many of the articles we used in research, so if you're keen to discover more, you might like to download that, too.

We hope reading this little book will feel like a chat with a good friend or a consultation with a particularly understanding GP – preferably both.

We wish you all the best on your journey.

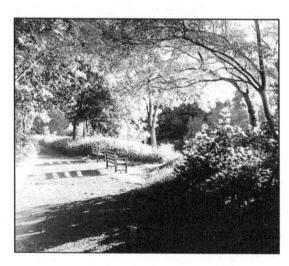

Contents

- Thinning hair
- Brittle nails
- Further unusual menopausal symptoms
- Communicating with your doctor
  - Q&A: How to get the most from a consultation with your GP

Hormone Replacement Therapy can stop, or at least slow down, the clock when it comes to the effects of the menopause. But is it right for you?
- What is Hormone Replacement Therapy?
- What are the benefits of HRT?
- What are the drawbacks?
- Weighing up the pros and cons
- Different types of HRT
  - Q&A: Bio-Identical Hormones
- The final decision is yours
- Coming off HRT
  - Q&A: Does HRT simply delay the onset of menopausal symptoms until you stop taking it?

From acupuncture to yoga – alternative approaches to mental and physical health through the menopause
- Pharmaceutical options to HRT
- The pros and cons of an alternative approach
  - What should you choose?
  - Working with your body
  - More time
  - Finding a reputable practitioner
- Herbal remedies
  - A word of caution
  - What to look for
- Traditional Chinese Medicine

- Acupuncture
- Cognitive Behavioural Therapy
- Mindfulness meditation
- Yoga and Pilates
- Alexander Technique
- Massage

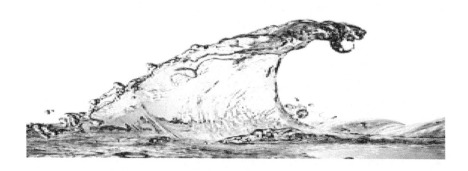

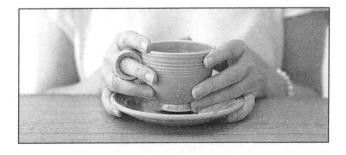

Introduction

0.1 Investing in your own wellbeing

'I just haven't the *time* to read a book on the menopause,' you might say, and I know where you're coming from. Even in relatively privileged western societies many women are concerned about daily survival and don't feel they have the headspace to think deeply about the menopause. In mid-life we're often faced with other issues: more than 1 million people in the UK are part of the 'sandwich generation', stuck in the middle supporting elderly parents and older children: in America over 1 in 8 of those aged 40-60 are both raising a child and caring for a parent.

'The menopause has increased my anxiety and lack of memory, and I find it harder to make decisions,' says Janet, a member of *Making Friends with the Menopause* on Facebook. 'This has made it hard to carry on with my job. I think there are now more women experiencing these physical and mental changes with careers than there were in our mothers' time.' Janet's experience is not unusual, and when we're juggling family commitments with work and are feeling unwell to boot, further demands can seem a burden, especially when so many books on the menopause are weighty and intimidating. Research shows an ostrich-like reaction to the subject is very common, and whilst I acknowledge that no one likes to focus on discomfort and distress, doesn't that strike you as curious? After all, what other major physical change do women go through that causes so many of us to bury our heads in the sand?

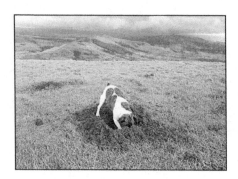

Not *starting* menstruating, for sure. When my periods began, I recall telling my female school friends in an excited whisper that I'd 'come on', and discussions about boyfriends and losing our virginity were had with equal verve. Educational achievements, job successes and disappointments, getting married or choosing not to, having or not having children – we even prepare for retirement and death with pensions and funeral plans. **Different cultural backgrounds mean we mark these changes in a multitude of ways,** nonetheless these physical and emotional transitions are discussed and dissected, celebrated and commiserated over.

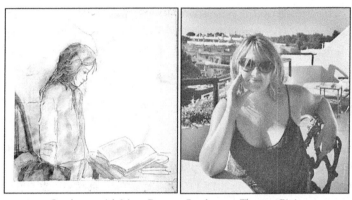

Sarah as a girl, Mary Rayner; Sarah now, Thomas Bicât

Yet talking about the menopause remains almost taboo, and for men broaching the topic can be even harder. The result is that this shift from one stage of our lives to another frequently remains shrouded in mystery until we find ourselves right in the middle of it, floundering and unsure.

*'Most women live to go through this transition. Many struggle. I did not want to be pronounced sick or judged as a hypochondriac; I just wanted to be told that what I was experiencing was normal and given advice about how to deal with it. I learned more from reading **Making Friends with the Menopause** and being in the affiliated support group than anywhere else, and I am now managing well with a combination of lifestyle changes and homeopathic remedies, but I wonder how many days of work are lost and how*

many false diagnoses are the result of the ignorance of medics and their failure to offer support and sensible advice?' **Mary, 52**

80% of women going through the menopause experience some symptoms – that's 1.5 million women in the UK at any one time. It's a strange contradiction: on one hand the menopause, after starting our periods, is the most universal physical experience of a woman's life (given not all women have children). On the other hand, it's one of the least talked about! In the face of such collective denial, perhaps it's unsurprising that it's taken until very recently for GPs to be given any formal guidance as to treatments. NICE was set up in 1999 in order to make 'evidence-based recommendations for health and care in England', and there are agreements in place so that the findings are available to those in the rest of the UK. Yet it wasn't until November 2015 that a press release aptly entitled 'NICE issues first guideline on menopause to stop women suffering in silence' heralded the publication of the guidelines which appraised the clinical options available.

'Every woman who is worried about the effects that menopause is having on her life must be given the chance to find if there's an option that works for her,' says Professor Lumsden, chair of the expert group which developed the NICE guidelines. I agree wholeheartedly with this sentiment, because whilst I don't expect every menopausal woman to run up a flag announcing to the neighbours that her periods have finished, I *do* believe that **knowledge is power.**

Making Friends with the Menopause can be read in a few hours, which is not a huge outlay of time when weighed against the years it takes to journey through the menopause. It doesn't aim to cover every symptom in detail but it *does* aim to provide an overview of the main changes your body goes through. Very few women sail through the menopause with no issues at all, so it's worth persevering as you could save yourself a great deal of discomfort and upset in the long run.

0.2 What exactly *is* the menopause?

The word 'menopause' stems from *men*, the Greek word for 'month', and *pausis*, meaning 'stop'.

The Concise Oxford Dictionary definition of 'menopause' is 'the cessation of the menses' and it has been noted the word has negative associations. It focuses attention on stopping, writes Bonnie J. Horrigan in *Red Moon Passage,* silently inferring nothing exists beyond that end. Author Lisa Jey Davis says she calls it "Orchids" because menopause is such an ugly word; it has '"men" in it for godsake'.

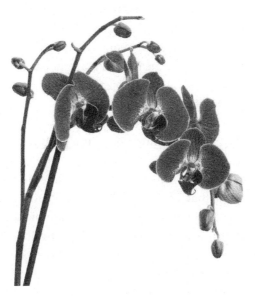

If 'menopause' is taken as the end of menstruation, in a literal sense it only lasts a day. But most of us don't think about it that way. Webster's Dictionary gives a secondary meaning; menopause is 'the whole group of physical and physiological changes that occur in the menopausal woman', and Farlax Medical Dictionary clarifies: 'While technically it refers to the final period, it is not an abrupt event, but a gradual process.'

Evidently the definition 'menopause' is not written in stone. No definition ever is. Words change in meaning throughout time and have different connotations for each of us.

0.3 Do men have a menopause, too?

Often we hear talk of a male menopause, whether there is one, and what symptoms it has. The etymology of the word 'menopause' permits us to nip this notion in the bud right now. '**Menopause' means 'cessation of the menses'** and/or the physical and physiological changes around this occurrence, and **last time I heard, men didn't have periods.** Ergo, men don't experience a menopause. **Men can have an 'andropause',** when they go through a drop in hormones and may experience other changes, both physical and mental. But in women, ovulation ends and hormone production plummets during a relatively short period of time. Whereas in men, hormone production and testosterone decline over a great many years and the consequences aren't necessarily clear. Biologically they are not the same, and men can't co-opt our experience. If the subject interests you, there is further reading listed at the end.

0.4 How society views the menopause – as a problem

Now we've sorted that out, let's return to the matter in hand.

It's interesting that as well as being hard to speak about, the words we tend to use when we *do* talk about the menopause are ones which we wouldn't use so readily about other physical life changes. In particular, **we talk about 'symptoms' of the menopause and 'treatment' for those symptoms**. Yet we don't tend to talk about 'symptoms' of adolescence or 'treatments' for puberty. Given that the primary definition of a 'symptom' in Webster's is 'evidence of disease', this suggests that our society views the menopause as an illness or dysfunction. And although Farlax reminds readers that **'the menopause is not a disease that needs to be cured, but a natural life-stage transition'**, it still seems we believe that being menopausal means something is *wrong* with us.

Women's health educator Magnolia Miller points out in her blog on **www.healthline.com** that this linguistic association heralds from the 1930s and 40s, which is when hormone treatment was first made available in the U.S. She believes its origins lie in marketing communication from drug companies who needed to create demand for their products.

It's also striking that there is no word for 'menopause' in some languages. In Japanese the closest word is 'konenki', which describes 'a transition in terms of lived experience', rather than focusing on the cessation of menstruation. Does this mean Japanese women don't experience the menopause? Of course their periods stop like the rest of us. But it appears significant that in a culture which tends to revere old age, they use a word with very different emphasis.

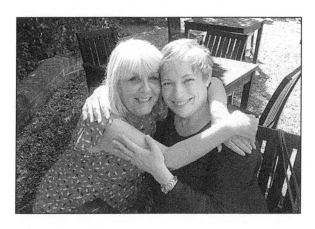

Perhaps you feel all these are only words and don't matter much. But trust that I draw attention to these issues not merely to nitpick, but because I believe **how the society we live in views the menopause has a huge impact on how we view** *ourselves*.

0.5 How we might view the menopause instead – as a natural life transition

We can't divest ourselves of this cultural baggage by leaving it in Left Luggage, and I have to write within the confines of the English language, so I've used words like 'symptom' and 'treatment' where alternatives sounded forced. Nonetheless I feel – as does Patrick – that **it's far more helpful and healing to see the menopause as rich with both negative** *and* **positive meaning, and that a more nuanced view will enable each of us to make a 'friend' of our individual experience overall.**

Part of that experience is ceasing periods and saying goodbye to our fertility, which means the menopause is a kind of spiritual and emotional ending that can involve intense feelings of anger and sorrow. But **the menopause is a new beginning too; a time when our sense of meaning and purpose in life as women can change enormously**. It's a psychological watershed – both a return to girlhood and a shift forward into maturity – and an opportunity for transformation and growth.

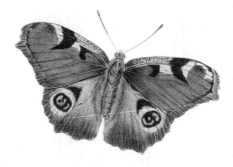

'We must become the change we want to see.' **Mahatma Gandhi**

1.   'M' is for Menstruation

Let's begin by looking at the origins of the menopause in terms of biology. What, physically, is its trigger? This should help us understand more fully what's happening in our bodies.

1.1 The role of hormones in our reproductive cycle

Remember that I said this book was a bit like doing a GSCE in the menopause? Well, it's a long time since I studied biology, and I suspect the same may be true for many of you, dear readers, so here comes the 'science bit'. The menstrual cycle is a recurring process, taking around 28 days. During this time, the lining of the womb is prepared for pregnancy, and if pregnancy does not happen, the lining is then shed.

This process is controlled by certain hormones. Hormones are your body's chemical messengers, which travel in your bloodstream to tissues or organs. They're essential for everyday life – for digestion and growth, for mood control and, in this case, for reproduction. Our reproductive hormones regulate certain cells and organs and are secreted by the ovaries and pituitary gland. During the menstrual cycle:

- **Follicle Stimulating Hormone (FSH)** is released by the pituitary gland.
  - It causes an egg to mature in an ovary
  - It stimulates the ovaries to release the hormone oestrogen
- **Oestrogen** (sometimes referred to as 'estrogen') is secreted by the ovaries. Oestrogen makes two things happen:
  - It stops FSH being produced so that only one egg matures in a cycle
  - It stimulates the pituitary gland to release the Luteinizing Hormone (LH)
- **Luteinizing Hormone** causes the mature egg to be released from the ovary.

21

- **Progesterone** is a hormone secreted by ovaries. It maintains the lining of the uterus during the middle part of the menstrual cycle and throughout pregnancy.

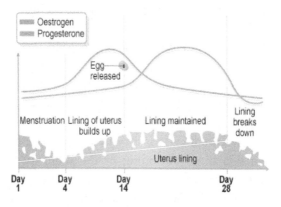

Hormone levels during the menstrual cycle ©BBC.co.uk

So far, so good, but of course we're not here to talk about our fertile years as such, we're focusing on the years around when the 'meno' (our cycle) 'pauses'.

There are three commonly recognised phases to the menopause, and each one is used to describe a different part of our journey and associated with different physical effects.

- Premenopause, also called the 'perimenopause'
- Menopause
- Postmenopause

Let's start with the first of these.

1.2 The perimenopause – the phase when hormone levels fluctuate

'I hadn't given even a second's thought to the possibility that in my early forties I would be a candidate – in my ignorance, I thought the menopause was something that happened to women in their mid-fifties, so I hadn't invested any time in learning about the menopausal phases and associated 'symptoms' of each one, which meant they crept up on me. The menopause wasn't a

subject that was discussed with other female friends beforehand – it didn't seem relevant to us at the time. The various conditions that I've experienced since, such as heart palpitations, hip joint pains, irritability, hairs appearing in places I never knew I even had follicles and days of inexplicable fatigue (to name but a few), I explained away under the generic umbrella of "getting older" and, in the case of my mood shifts, the vagaries of my personality. The heart palpitations did alarm me though, so I had that checked out and was relieved to find that it was nothing sinister. Even then no one mentioned that I could be perimenopausal.' **Chloe, 48**

The perimenopause is the transition period leading up to the menopause and signifies the winding down of the ovaries. But the ovaries rarely suddenly shut up shop; instead **fertility declines gradually**.

- During perimenopause, levels of oestrogen fluctuate and become unpredictable. Eventually, production falls to a very low level.
- Progesterone production stops after the final menstrual period.
- This fall in hormones affects every aspect of a woman's body, from sex drive to brain function.
- High levels of oestrogen can result in bloating, breast tenderness and heavy bleeding.
- Low levels of oestrogen can result in hot flushes (known as hot 'flashes' in America and Canada), night sweats, palpitations, insomnia and vaginal dryness.
- Lack of progesterone can cause periods to become irregular, heavier and longer during perimenopause.
- Many women find the physical effects intensify as the decline in oestrogen accelerates.
- The mean age of perimenopausal onset is 47.5 years. Approximately 10% of women find their periods come to an abrupt halt, but in most women going through a natural menopause, this phase usually lasts about four years.
- Occasionally perimenopause can be far longer (up to ten years).
- In women who have undergone gynaecological surgery or certain medical treatments, the transition tends to occur more quickly.

23

- During the perimenopause it's still possible to become pregnant, so you should use contraception if you don't wish to conceive. Let's look into this in a little more detail.

Contraception during the perimenopause and menopause

As long as you are having periods you are fertile – even when your periods have stopped you can remain fertile for another year. **If you are sexually active and don't wish to conceive, it's important to remember contraception.**

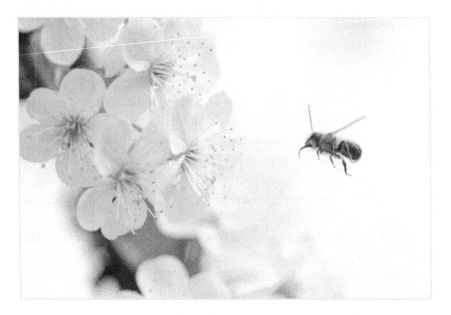

Q&A

Sarah: What contraception would you advise women to use? What are the most common side effects?

Patrick: Each woman will have her own preference. Some like daily tablets, others the ease of the coil. All methods are open to use, but there are caveats depending on side effects and whether or not HRT is used at the same time. The Faculty of Sexual and Reproductive Health recently issued guidance for 'older women' which readers can find at https://www.fsrh.org/news/updated-clinical-guideline-published-contraception-for-women/. Here's a brief overview of their recommendations:

1. Combined Oral Contraception (COC). It used to be that patients were advised to stop taking this common form of the pill around 40. Now the guidance says you can continue until you are 50, but you shouldn't continue on COC over the age of 35 if you:

- Smoke
- Are overweight
- Have heart disease/high blood pressure or high cholesterol

This is because COC can increase the risk of cardiac events and blood clots. On the plus side, the oestrogen in COC can help to alleviate menopausal symptoms, which means you are unlikely to need HRT, and certain pills (such as Qlaira) offer a shorter breakthrough bleed of only two days. This is very helpful if you suffer from heavy menstrual bleeding.

2. Progesterone Only Pill (POP) – commonly called the 'mini pill'. This is taken every day and is safe to use until your periods stop. You can also use HRT at the same time, though the POP dose is often reduced.

3. Progesterone Implant (Nexplanon) and Depot Injection. Both methods use long-acting versions of progesterone but with the ease of not having to remember to take pills. As with the POP, having progesterone in your system means that your periods can stop, and side effects include spotting between periods, heavier bleeding, skin changes and mood alteration. There is no known link with reproductive cancers with progesterone alone, and it may be protective in endometrial cancer.

4. Intrauterine Device (IUD) or Coil. There are two kinds, copper and progesterone-coated. Copper coils are non-hormonal so can be used easily alongside HRT. However they are limited by their side effects, most notably heavy bleeding. Hormonal coils - Mirena, Levosert and Jaydess - are all licensed to use as contraceptive devices. The length of use varies according to the product but the Mirena is the only coil licensed for use with HRT so tends to be recommended first line:

- It is well tolerated
- It lasts five years
- Oral or topical oestrogen (HRT) can be added to control menopausal symptoms

Disadvantages include erratic bleeding, though this tends to settle over time, pain on intercourse, and – rarely – uterine pain. Don't forget that the Mirena needs replacing every 5 years – easy to forget! Put the date in your diary.

Sarah: How do women know when to stop using contraception?

Patrick: The general advice is that it is safe to stop contraception when you haven't had a period for over a year or are over 55. However, if you are taking the POP or using a Mirena coil, you may not have periods and won't be able to tell. In this scenario the FSH blood test can help confirm if you are post-menopausal.

Please remember that **this advice on contraception is general**. Your GP is best placed to tailor contraception to your needs. Alternatively, your local family planning clinic can provide guidance, (https://www.fpa.org.uk/find-a-clinic) and can also insert and remove coils.

Alternatively, if becoming pregnant is your goal, there are fertility-enhancing treatments that can help, although conception is never guaranteed. If you are in this position, you might find it helpful to read the sister book to this one: *Making Friends with your Fertility*, which is a more fulsome guide to reproductive health supporting you through the highs and lows of getting pregnant, IVF and assisted conception.

What happens to menstruation in perimenopause?

Some women find their periods become closer together, others further apart; some find blood flow is more scant, others more profuse. A lot of women have a mix of all these.

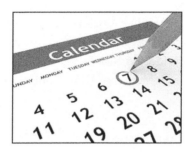

'I don't know where I am one month to the next.' **Janet, 51**

None of these fluctuations in your cycle indicate anything is necessarily 'wrong' physically – chances are it's just your body making the transition. Levels of hormones vary and may be higher or lower than normal during any cycle. If you don't ovulate one month – which is common for women in perimenopause – progesterone isn't produced to stimulate menstruation, and oestrogen levels continue to rise. This can cause spotting throughout your cycle or heavy bleeding when menstruation does start.

- If you are experiencing severe cramps, painkillers such as ibuprofen or paracetamol may provide relief.
- Erratic bleeding may be a sign of other problems, so do consult your doctor if you are at all worried.

'I don't think this stage of life is discussed enough and bleeding problems are rarely mentioned – everyone just talks about hot flushes. For me the worst symptom is the heavy and unpredictable periods. My social life is suffering because of it.' **Theresa, 48**

When irregular periods are NOT caused by the perimenopause

Sometimes irregular periods are not a result of the menopause. If you've ruled out being pregnant, the most common reasons for missed, irregular or heavy periods are:

- Stress
- A change in diet – sudden weight loss can have an impact on your periods
- The IUD (coil) – sometimes this causes spotting mid-cycle
- A change in medication – some medications (notably birth control pills) interfere with how your body produces oestrogen and progesterone which can make your period earlier or later than usual
- Excessive exercise
- An over- or under-active thyroid
- Fibroids
- Endometriosis
- Polycystic Ovary Syndrome (PCOS)

Q&A

Sarah: When are irregular periods a cause to worry?

Patrick: Age has a lot to do with it. As a rule of thumb I'd say if you are over 45, it is more likely that irregular periods are a sign that you're perimenopausal, but if you are under 45 and your periods have been regular and become noticeably heavier, or your cycle changes or you experience spotting mid-cycle, it's worth checking that there isn't another cause such as fibroids. But whatever your age, please don't panic – other causes of erratic periods are rarely life-threatening. Your doctor can discuss your level of physical discomfort and check if there is likely to be any impact on your fertility. Both can be treated, and your GP may well refer you to a gynecologist (a specialist in women's reproductive issues). However if you're bleeding between periods or after sex, I'd say go and see your doctor, although if your periods are erratic, I appreciate it can be hard to tell where you are in your cycle. Still, it's important to get checked out. This is what your GP is there for.

Sarah: Can my doctor test to see if I'm in the early stages of the menopause?

Patrick: Menopausal symptoms such as flushes and altered periods may be enough for your GP to suspect menopause. You don't have to have a blood test, and if you're over 45 you probably don't need one. For help with uncertainty your GP may want to test your FSH level amongst other tests such as thyroid function. However FSH results aren't 100% reliable because fluctuations of hormones are part and parcel of the experience. The combined pill will alter results too. Confusing!

It's even more difficult to know what stage you're at if you're taking the combined pill as that may mask signs your hormone levels are dropping. NICE say the FSH test should not be used to diagnose menopause in women using the combined oestrogen and progestogen pill as contraception, or high-dose progestogen as diagnostic accuracy may be confounded by these treatments.

In most cases I find that, just as NICE recommend, an assessment of symptoms tends to be the most useful gauge. If you're having menopausal symptoms that worry you, do seek advice from your GP. There's a *Test Yourself* Chart on **www.netdoctor.com** which should provide a good basis for discussion before you go.

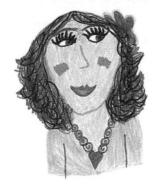 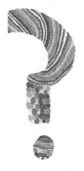

Illustration: Rosie Rayner

Sarah: While we're on the subject of the NICE guidelines, can you summarise what they are advising doctors?

Patrick: As a GP, I'm glad to get advice around menopause management, as there have been a lot of mixed messages over the years from different researchers. What's good about NICE is that the team review all the available evidence and weigh it up over many months before producing the guidance.

The guidance splits into diagnosis, management, and a section on premature ovarian failure which we're not covering in this book. In terms of diagnosis, I've just mentioned the main change, which is that for women with altered periods and clear menopausal symptoms over the age of 45, a blood test is no longer needed to diagnose potential menopause, as it's the most likely explanation, although there will naturally be circumstances where blood tests will help rule out other causes.

In terms of management, the biggest change is that the guidance states clearly that HRT is the best treatment for unmanageable menopausal symptoms. Yes, there is potential risk in terms of breast and endometrial cancer, but this risk needs to be looked at on an individual basis.

For those without a uterus, oestrogen-only HRT use is obligatory, and it seems to have a lower risk profile than combined HRT. For those with a uterus, the combination of topical oestrogen with a localised endometrial progestogen delivered by an IUCD, such as a Mirena coil, as discussed earlier in this chapter, may offer the lowest risk from combined HRT usage. I think it gives doctors more leeway to consider HRT as first-line treatment – something we'll return to in more detail in Chapter 5.

NICE's own summary of the guidelines can be found at www.nice.org.uk/guidance/ng23.

'I used to have very regular periods. I have endometriosis and, given the symptoms and pain that come with that, the regularity of my periods was a godsend because it meant I could plan around that week. I knew not to work too hard, not to have meetings or do too much that was important, and I

learned never to shop because I couldn't make proper decisions. But once I became perimenopausal, my periods became completely erratic. Sometimes it's two weeks between them, then five, then three, then two months...So I can't plan, which makes my work life really difficult, because I still get a similar amount of pain, and often the bleeding is heavier, so then I've been flattened. But then my last period was only five days and much lighter, which was completely disorientating.' **Holly, 54**

Common physical indicators of the perimenopause

As we've just mentioned, most of the impact on our bodies is caused by fluctuating levels of oestrogen and progesterone.

- Hot flushes
- Night Sweats
- Joint aches
- Nerve sensitivity
- Hair thinning (head, pubic or whole body, but increased facial hair)
- Weight gain
- Memory loss
- Difficulty concentrating and disorientation
- Loss of energy
- Tiredness
- Insomnia
- Headaches
- Vaginal dryness and thinning
- Loss of sexual desire
- Incontinence especially when sneezing and laughing

Many women notice these physical changes kick in during perimenopause and continue during menopause, after their periods have ceased.

'The impact of perimenopause was a shock. We tend to think of the menopause as stopping bleeding, but the run up can take years, and there's so much else

going on and it's really confusing. I felt like I didn't know who I was, and I still get that feeling now.' **Annie, 50**

'The trouble with the menopause is that we've no idea how far we are through the process. It's a journey where we don't know where we are or when it's going to end.' **Juliet, 53**

Common psychological effects of perimenopausal hormone change:

- Mood swings
- Heightened anxiety and panic attacks
- Sudden tears and depression
- Irritability and anger
- General dissatisfaction with life

If you've not thought much about the menopause until now, I can understand if these lists make uncomfortable reading. But they are not intended to cause dismay – quite the opposite. Often we may not realize what we're feeling is linked to the menopause and can find ourselves in serious discomfort, worrying we are going to be this way *indefinitely*. That was my fear, anyway, when it came to anxiety – I'd been anxious before, so who was to say having it badly wasn't just the way I was destined to be for the rest of my days? Moreover, many of these symptoms are quite nebulous – 'loss of energy' for instance, or 'difficulty concentrating' – and they may come and go, which means they are hard to gauge and describe to others.

It can also make it hard for us to trust ourselves and what we are feeling. That's not to say we shouldn't listen to our bodies or pay attention to these changes. **It can be an immense relief to discover there is a 'cause'** if our nerve endings seem as if they are on fire, or we experience panic attacks for the first time **and often this understanding can be a solace in itself**. Certainly it was a comfort to me.

'No one warned me how horrendous perimenopause could be. There isn't enough information – I actually thought I had dementia at one point. The impact it has had on my life – I had to give up work – cannot be over-

exaggerated. Knowing others had been through similar helped me to feel normal.' **Lynda, 47**

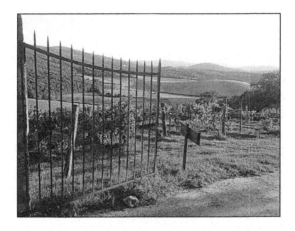

The knowledge your symptoms may well be linked to menopause can also be a gateway to seeking help. We'll look into these physical and psychological changes in more detail in ourselves and what we're feeling in the following chapters, and discuss options for managing them, including Hormone Replacement Therapy (HRT).

What is an early menopause?

There are many reasons for experiencing your menopause when you are younger than average. Sometimes our fertility starts to decline in our forties or, more rarely, in our thirties.

- If you experience the menopause between the ages of 40 and 45 and it is not medically or surgically initiated, you are said to be experiencing an 'early menopause'.
- Premature ovarian failure (POF) occurs when the ovaries slow or stop production of mature eggs and reproductive hormones before the age of 40. Roughly one woman in every 100 begins her menopause by the age of 35.

Although population studies have shown that family history, smoking and low socio-economic factors make the likelihood of an early menopause higher, in 70% of individual cases the cause remains unknown.

Early menopause can also arise as a result of surgery or drug regimes:

- Surgical menopause is a result of a hysterectomy, removal of ovaries and other pelvic surgeries. Ablations (procedures to remove the lining of the uterus) can mimic menopause by stopping menstrual periods. If your ovaries are removed during a hysterectomy, you will go through the menopause immediately after the operation, regardless of your age. If one or both of your ovaries remain intact, you are likely to experience the menopause within five years of having your operation.
- Medical menopause may occur after treatments such as chemotherapy or radiation therapy, and as a result of drug treatments – tamoxifen, which is used primarily to prevent the reoccurrence of breast cancer, is one example.

The emotional impact of early menopause

No matter what led to your experiencing an early menopause, **it's very understandable to feel shocked and upset.**

'I was diagnosed with breast cancer at 41. Following a harrowing six months of surgery, then chemotherapy, I was put on tamoxifen. The cancer was gone but it pushed me straight into the perimenopause, with mood swings and night sweats. I also got depressed – I was coming to terms with the cancer, with the treatment and with the way my body was changing as a result of the tamoxifen suppressing my oestrogen. I am prone to depression – I had my first severe episode at 18, and then every few years since – but this one was bad, and I had to take time off work.' **Vicky, 52**

'My menopause began when I was 40 but I didn't find out I was perimenopausal until I tried to have another child. I had tests to find out why I wasn't getting pregnant and discovered I had a low egg count, which was very upsetting and stressful.' **Annie, 42**

Many women, learning they are in premature menopause, ask 'why me?' and worry about what may have caused it and what it means for their future.

- Early menopause can be a blow to your self-esteem, making you feel powerless and older than your age.
- Some women feel they have lost their womanhood. These feelings are common among women of all ages going through menopause and is a subject we return to later.
- If you haven't yet had children and wanted to, the grief of discovering you are experiencing an early menopause can be even more intense.

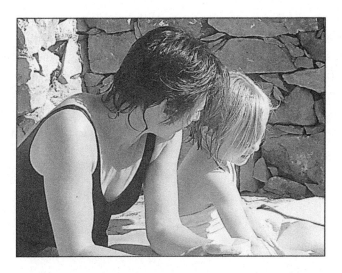

The path to motherhood is not always what we plan, but that does not mean that we will never be mothers. Because fertility tends to decline gradually not suddenly, some women who are experiencing an early menopause (between 5-10%) do manage to become pregnant without medical intervention and prior to oophorectomy (removal of the ovaries), egg freezing may be a possibility. In most cases, egg donation is the most likely route to pregnancy.

No matter whether you're experiencing a natural or induced early menopause, **it's important to consider if you wish to reduce the**

physical impact of hormonal change. It's possible that when you have supports in place to relieve the physical transition, your emotional health will not suffer as greatly. The most common treatment offered in these circumstances is HRT – see Chapter 5. Whatever your situation, **if you are experiencing the menopause before you expected to, I would encourage you to seek additional emotional support to help work through some of the emotions associated with its arrival.**

'What is wrong with her, with her womb, with her ability to mother, that makes her incapable of nurturing life? She rubs her belly. "Forgive me," she says.'

Sarah Rayner, extract from **The Two Week Wait**

You may feel you need to let go of the previous woman you were and that can be difficult. But remember that menopause can be a time of reflection and insight, and when you are through the mourning process (in so far as one is ever 'through' with grieving), your life's journey will continue.

'Sometimes the things we can't change end up changing us.' **Anonymous**

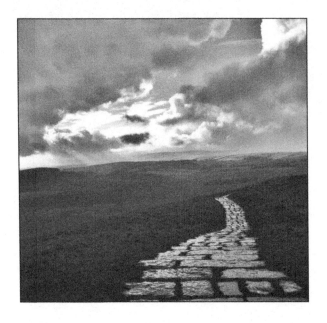

1.3 The menopause – the phase straight after your last period

Eventually the ovaries no longer produce eggs. Monthly periods stop and fertility ceases. **The average age that periods cease for women in the UK and USA is 51.**

My periods finally ground to a halt at 49, but the problem was I didn't *know* it was my last period when it happened – if I had I might have thrown a little party! – and, (unless you've psychic powers worthy of Mystic Meg) nor will you. This only compounds the whole nebulous sense of the menopause, which is defined as the 12 months after your last period. If your menstrual cycle has been winding down gradually, as mine did, it's pretty likely you'll go from having a period every few weeks, to stopping, and not realize. I still couldn't tell you when my last period was, even now – just that I stopped about two or three years ago, and I bet I'm not alone in this.

Moreover, whilst the average age of menopause is 51, it's just an average. I've friends of 53 and 54 who still menstruate. When my periods started it was similar: some of my classmates had their first period at 12-years-old, others at 16. Factors that can affect when an individual has her final period include the age of menarche (when she had her first period), previous oral contraceptive history, smoking, Body Mass Index (BMI), ethnicity, family history, and a history of breast surgery.

Many women find that the physical changes they first noticed in the perimenopause intensify during menopause – though often, for the reasons I've outlined, we may not be able to see this clearly until after the fact.

According to Consultant Gynecologist, Mr Haitham Hamoda, 80-90% of women experience symptoms after their periods have stopped. Hot flushes, for instance, the most widely-experienced and obvious physical indictor of menopause, are experienced by well over half of menopausal women. Again, I'd emphasize this isn't a cause for despair – the good news is the menopause doesn't last forever.

Donna Fedorkow, Professor of Obstetrics and Gynecology at McMaster University believes that 95% of us will stop having symptoms within five years of our last period. New evidence suggests it can go on longer, particularly for Afro-Caribbean women, and so for a small but significant minority hot flushes will continue, but for most women, the majority of symptoms, including hot flushes and night sweats, will go within two years.

'I talk about the menopause a lot with friends of the same age, but younger friends don't understand. Until you experience it, you've no idea what it feels like.' **Juliet, 53**

'Menopause seems to be seen by most people as a bit of a joke. Until it happens to you – then it's not so funny.' **Shelley, 51**

<u>Q&A</u>

Sarah: When should I seek medical advice? I never know whether I should just put up with the physical effects of menopause because I'm only going through what every other woman does – hot flushes are so common, after all – or if I should go to my doctor. What guidance would you give?

Patrick: Whether you choose to seek treatment or wait until your hormones settle is down to each person. What matters is the level of concern these physical and psychological changes are causing you. Ask yourself: How **disturbed** am I by what I am feeling? Am I **coping** or not coping? Am I in **serious pain** or more mild discomfort?

Taking your hot flushes as an example, if they are accompanied by night sweats, does this mean you can't sleep and are tired at work all day? Or is it more a case that you wake up hot and sticky, but generally rested? I'd say the level of concern is greater if the answer to the first question is yes, and a consultation with your GP could be helpful, as there are medications which can help. If you're finding you can still sleep well – given you know the cause is likely to be hormonal and thus a normal physical reaction related to this time in your life – perhaps you can wait and see if the experience gets better of its own accord. If it worsens, then take action. I'd recommend trying some of the lifestyle changes featured in the following chapters first.

1.4 Postmenopause – 12 months after your last period and beyond

Just as it's hard to define when we're menopausal, it's also hard to define exactly when we're postmenopausal. In her book *New Menopausal Years, The Wise Woman Way*, Susun S.

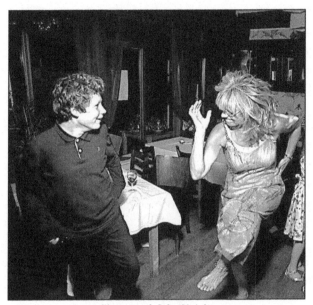

Photograph John Knight

Weed defines it as 14 months after your last period. More usually it's said to be when a woman hasn't bled or spotted for 12 months, as we've mentioned. In any event, **this means we are no longer ovulating and capable of conceiving a child.**

Whilst menopausal indicators such as hot flushes tend to ease off after menopause, postmenopausal women are at increased risk of a number of health conditions such as osteoporosis and heart disease as a result of a lower level of oestrogen. This does not mean your body stops making sex hormones altogether – but it does mean you almost certainly won't get pregnant. So let's not underestimate the **positive physical and psychological changes that come as a result of the menopause too.** The cessation of a monthly bleed can be incredibly liberating – you can throw out those tampons and sanitary towels and buy yourself some nice new underwear for a start – and some women enjoy a burst of energy when they're out the other side.

'No more periods – what joy! I don't have children and had never desperately wanted them so wasn't worried about the end of my
fertility. Instead I was massively relieved to be free of all the hassle.' **Vicky, 52**

'Ah, the relief of knowing I have stopped having periods – forever. All that faffing with tampons and pads, making sure I didn't run out of painkillers, worrying about stains on my skirt – thank goodness it's over. I can wear white again!' **Juliet, 53**

- Fibroids usually stop growing and shrink when women reach menopause.
- After years of hiatus, it means the end of the guessing game as to what's happening and when, in your cycle.
- No longer being fertile means you can have sex without worrying about getting pregnant.

All this can be very liberating, and we'll return to the subject of life after the menopause in Chapter 7.

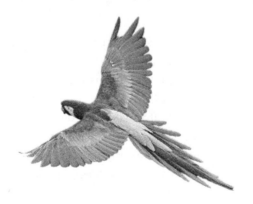

2. 'E' is for Emotion

So now we're more familiar with the three phases of the menopause and the physical changes associated with each stage, let's take a closer look at how this transition can affect our moods.

I'd like to start by asking you to cast your mind back. Do you remember being a teenager? How (if you were anything like me) you veered from anger and despair to laughter and happiness on an almost hourly basis? Your first kiss, your first love affair, your first holiday without your parents, your first driving lesson? These experiences are often burned into our memory, so intense were our feelings. Maybe you've got kids who've been through puberty, so you've been reminded more recently what an emotional see-saw it can be. Children who were once cooperative and a pleasure to be around are one minute grunting and disinterested in anything you say, the next holding you responsible for every ill on this planet.

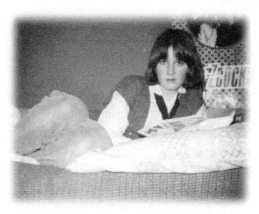

Sarah at 15

'Adolescence is a period of rapid changes. Between the ages of 12 and 17 a parent can age as much as 20 years.'

Anonymous

Whilst other factors can contribute to adolescent volatility, it's nonetheless the case that our reproductive hormones have a profound influence on our bodies and behaviour, and it's only when the brakes on oestrogen and testosterone are released that girls and boys begin to morph into adults. But whilst we're accustomed to seeing teenagers as the embodiment of hormonal mayhem, what's less widely acknowledged is that **the female body undergoes enormous chemical changes as a result of the menopause, and that this can also have a big impact on our emotions too**.

2.1 'Why do I feel OK one day and awful the next?' – Mood swings

We saw in the diagram at the beginning of Chapter 1 how much our hormones go up and down when we menstruate. These peaks and troughs can influence our moods long before menopause – hence premenstrual tension (PMT).

We then learned that our hormones can fluctuate in perimenopause. The result, for some women, is like PMT, but worse. Our moods can veer all over the shop, something doctors and psychologists tend to refer to as 'mood swings'. Personally, I feel that to say I was subject to 'mood swings' when I was perimenopausal is an understatement. 'Swings' sound too much fun. I'd call them 'mood crashes', myself. You don't have control in a car crash, and I certainly didn't feel I had control of my moods.

My problem was anxiety. My goodness, was it overwhelming. So overwhelming I had to cease work, I couldn't drive or socialise, and on many occasions I felt as if I was pinned to the floor by panic. For other women, the black dog of depression might bite at this time. Both are debilitating and distressing, and – especially if you've not suffered problems with your mental health hitherto – f rightening. There is little more terrifying an experience than losing the very sense of who you are. Other women may become irritable and angry, experience memory loss and have difficulty concentrating, or a combination of these.

Many so-called psychological symptoms of the menopause can be attributed to the known reduction of blood flow to the brain as oestrogen deprivation causes blood vessels to constrict. The result is clumsiness, a reduced reaction time and a lack of ability to judge distance, along with a woolly 'out of body' feeling. Sound familiar? I don't know about you, but it seems awfully like how I felt with PMT.

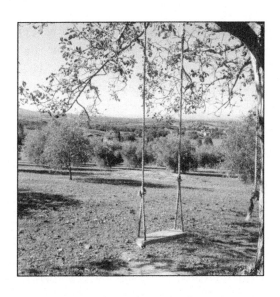

Unfortunately, when I was perimenopausal, I was unaware of the power of my hormones. Ignorance was *not* bliss; I grew more and more anxious. Eventually I got so desperate that I consulted a psychiatrist. Yet when I asked whether he thought my age (49) might have anything to do with how panicky I was feeling, he said that it was 'unlikely', pointing out that I had a history of being anxious. I told him my anxiety had got much worse, and I believed I was going through the menopause. 'My antidepressants don't seem to work like they used to,' I said. (I'd been on a maintenance dose for many years.) He agreed it was possible that they'd lost their efficacy and we switched my medication, which helped.

At the time I believed the psychiatrist knew best because he was an expert, but now I'm out the other side of the menopause, my moods have stabilised. This seems more than a coincidence, so I've looked into it more closely, and lo, I've discovered that panic disorder *is* common at this time. Stacey B Gramann, Psychiatry Resident at the University of Massachusetts, reports in a survey of nearly 3,500 women aged 50-79 years, panic attacks were most common among women in the menopause. It's a similar story with depression: investigators from the Harvard Study of Moods and Cycles recruited premenopausal women aged 36-44 years with no history of major depression. They then followed up these women for nine years to detect new onsets of major depression and – bingo! According to Gramann, they found that women who entered perimenopause were twice as likely to have clinically significant depressive symptoms as women who were as yet not perimenopausal.

So if I were sitting opposite *you* in a psych consultation and you asked if the menopause could be contributing to your fluctuating mood, I'd say, 'Yes, certainly.' Frankly, I wish the psychiatrist had said that to me back then. There might be other contributing factors, but **perimenopausal mood swings and crashes are also often linked to fluctuating oestrogen and progesterone levels**. It would have been comforting to know many women have felt the way I did at a similar time in their lives and that I was thus 'normal'. As I said earlier, my biggest fear was that the anxiety was going to be permanent, and this would have given me hope that it might not be. It's also possible I might have opted for HRT instead. Certainly I would have liked to have given it consideration.

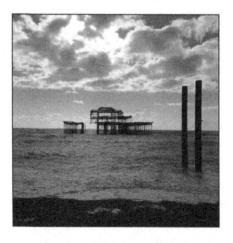

'Life always gives you a second chance. It's called tomorrow.' **Anonymous**

Of course I'm not your GP, or your psychiatrist, and there can be other physical causes of low mood than our fluctuating reproductive hormones. Thyroid issues affect how we feel emotionally too, for example, and can occur at any age. Nonetheless, **if you believe that**

44

you are perimenopausal and you feel more anxious, depressed, angry or irritable than before, the odds are your more intense emotional state *is* connected to the changes going on in your body. Same – or similar – to adolescence, then. Only, in our teens the brakes were coming off our reproductive hormones; during the perimenopause they are coming *on*.

Next, let's shine a light on the dark emotions of anxiety, depression and anger and learn more about tackling each one.

2.2 'I feel like I'm having a heart attack' – Anxiety

You don't need to be a medical expert to understand that your ovaries don't operate in a little world of their own down there in your abdomen. If you've ever felt physically attracted to someone else, it should be pretty clear that your reproductive organs are linked to your brain. **It's important to remember that our bodies and minds are connected if we're to make sense of how we feel during the menopause and learn how to manage our emotions more effectively**.

A shift in your hormone balance can create stress throughout your entire body. In Chapter 1 we learned how levels of both reproductive hormones fall as our ovaries shut down; this helps explain why women in perimenopause may feel more overwhelmed and easily stressed. **Lowering progesterone is one of the hallmarks of this time and can cause women to feel anxious, edgy, and short-tempered.** Progesterone acts as a natural sedative, softening and balancing the effects of oestrogen and promoting sleep.

Because progesterone is a woman's calming hormone, with less progesterone women may begin to feel more overwhelmed and easily stressed. In many women, this leads to anxiety issues, including tension headaches, palpitations, digestive issues and more – and, in some cases, full blown panic disorder.

In addition, alongside your body changes, you may well be experiencing other life events around the time of perimenopause which can exacerbate anxiety. As I approached 50, for instance, I became aware of my own mortality and a whole lot more besides. And in the case of anxiety, it's not all about oestrogen and progesterone – when we're stressed other hormones get involved too: most notably adrenaline.

The role of adrenaline

To understand adrenaline, we need to go back much further than our own lifespan and memory, to a time when humans had to hunt and forage for food. This is because **anxiety is the biological vestige of fear**, the basic survival mechanism that helps safeguard us against danger and threats such as predators. In this respect we could say that **adrenaline is a hormone that doesn't care if you've less progesterone in your system to temper its impact or not. It's got a job to do and it'll do it regardless.**

- When we experience fear **the brain sends a biochemical message which triggers the release of the stress hormone, adrenaline**.
- It's all systems go – **our breathing becomes faster and shallower,** supplying more oxygen to the muscles.
- **Our hearts beat more rapidly and blood is driven to the brain and limbs** so we can make split-second decisions and a quick getaway. This is why we experience heart palpitations, chest pains and tingling when we are afraid.
- **Blood is taken from areas of the body where it's not needed,** such as the stomach, because in a life-threatening situation, you're not going to stop for food. Thus when you're afraid, you may well feel sick and be unable to eat.
- **The liver releases stored sugar to provide fuel for quick energy.** Excess sugar in the blood can cause indigestion.
- **Muscles at the opening of the anus and bladder are relaxed.** Food and liquid are evacuated so you're lighter to run. Hence diarrhoea and frequent urination.
- **The body cools itself by perspiring.** Blood vessels and capillaries move close to the skin surface, leading to sweating and blushing.

You may well recognise these physical symptoms and suffer from a few, in which case it can be helpful to understand that they are linked to a normal biological reaction.

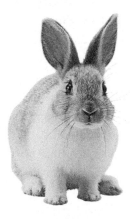

Animals have similar responses, which in itself can alleviate the fear there is something more serious wrong with us. Everyone experiences anxiety at some point, but when it becomes out of proportion, persistent or appears for no apparent reason, it can become a problem. What happens then is that adrenaline production is triggered in response to situations where we don't actually *need* to run away or fight for survival. In perimenopause, lessening progesterone can mean this happens more frequently, and if we experience this series of reactions in an unexpected environment such as in a supermarket or business meeting, it can be very frightening. If you can, the important thing to remind yourself when this occurs is that **none of the symptoms listed above are dangerous in themselves.**

'Before any change I was fit and able. The menopause took me and my family by surprise. I had debilitating anxiety and fear with every possible associated symptom. I looked for help, someone to talk to, people to understand without judgement. There are baby groups for new mothers and toddler groups but where are the menopause groups? Other than the Making Friends with the Menopause Facebook group, we have little to offer women. Some of us don't want antidepressants, we just want to be reassured and to see the light.'
Joanna, 52

Making Friends with Anxiety

If you're hyper anxious, it's unlikely you'll be able to settle down until the adrenaline subsides, but **the main secret to overcoming anxiety is not to fight it. We** *need* **fear, however horrible it feels to be afraid.**

When my anxiety was very bad, I fought it tooth and nail. Often I'd think I'd do anything to get rid of it; sometimes I'd even shout 'get out of my head!' and beat my own forehead. Once I'd got to grips with the role of adrenaline, it helped me change my attitude. I realized I *couldn't* switch anxiety off, however desperately I wanted to, because it was inextricably linked to fear. Gradually, I began to appreciate it was what had kept me alive. It was the start of making friends with my anxiety and the beginning of my road to recovery.

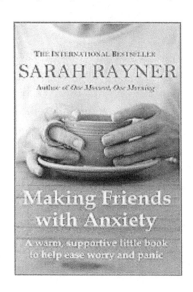

Dealing with panic attacks and raised anxiety alongside other menopausal symptoms can be particularly hard, so if you're finding it difficult to manage, you might like to read *Making Friends with Anxiety,* which provides a fuller explanation and tips centring around using Mindfulness-Based Cognitive Behaviour Therapy. You could also join the *Making Friends with Anxiety & Depression* support group online. It has nearly 10,000 members and sharing experiences with people may well help ease your fears. (There's nothing to stop you joining it as well as the *Making Friends with the Menopause* group. Many women are in both.) You can find the group – which is 'closed' so private - at www.facebook.com/groups/makingfriendswithanxiety/

*TIP: 'When I feel anxiety rising, I gently tell myself that much of what I'm experiencing is because of adrenaline and there's no need to be afraid. I suggest you try similar: act normally if you can, and accept that it will pass. Remind yourself it's **only** anxiety, **only** adrenaline, and that in itself it can't harm you.'* **Sarah Rayner, Making Friends with Anxiety**

Interestingly NICE now recommend the consideration of HRT and CBT for menopause-related symptoms. We'll look further into HRT in Chapter 5, and CBT in Chapter 6.

2.3 'I'm so low, I could crawl under the carpet and stay there' – Depression

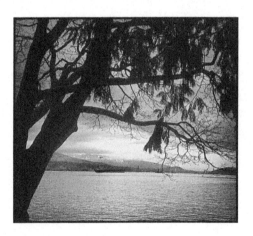

'How weary, stale, flat and unprofitable,
Seem to me all the uses of this world!'
                    William Shakespeare, extract from **Hamlet**

When we're discussing depression, **it's important to make the distinction between being unhappy and being clinically depressed from the outset**. The latter is a physical illness with many more symptoms than an unhappy mood.

Sadness:

- Feeling sad as a result of painful circumstances is part of the human condition
- Sadness is a transient feeling that passes when we come to terms with these circumstances
- When we are sad we feel bad, but continue to cope with living

Depression:

- If you are suffering from depression, you often can't find a logical reason for your low mood
- Depression can linger for weeks, months or even years
- You may well feel overwhelmed by life and hopeless about the future

Although the majority of women go through the menopause without becoming clinically depressed, **an estimated 20% experience depression at some point. Like anxiety, studies of mood reveal that risk tends to be highest during the perimenopause**, with a decrease in risk during postmenopausal years. If you believe you might be suffering from depression, the main signs to look for are:

- A profound lack of energy, motivation and drive. Tasks which previously seemed straightforward become monumentally difficult
- Markedly diminished pleasure in all, or most, daily activities, nearly every day
- Significant weight changes or decrease or increase in appetite nearly every day
- Insomnia or hypersomnia (sleeping too much) nearly every day
- Excessive or inappropriate guilt nearly every day
- Indecisiveness or diminished ability to think or concentrate nearly every day
- Loss of self-worth and self-esteem
- Occasional agoraphobia and claustrophobia
- Recurrent thoughts of death or suicide

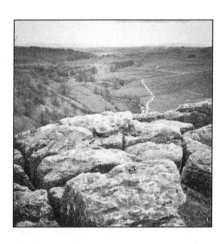

'Nothing is so painful to the human mind as a great and sudden change.'
Mary Shelley, extract from **Frankenstein**

It can be very hard to diagnose yourself, especially if you're feeling extremely low. Moreover **depression and anxiety often go hand in hand,** so it's quite possible you may lurch from one to the other.

Much as I'd love to wave a magic wand and cure your depression, it can be a life-threatening illness, so it would be irresponsible of me to claim that I can ease anyone's anguish in a couple of paragraphs. And whilst there is evidence that hormone changes in menopause – in particular the decline in oestrogen – can contribute to depression and that Hormone Replacement Therapy can relieve emotional symptoms linked to menopause, HRT alone is not proven to be effective in treating more severe depression.

In addition, alongside your body changes, you may well be experiencing other life events around the time of perimenopause which can have a big impact on your mood – children leaving home, or the infirmity or passing of elder family members, for instance. When it comes to managing a complex mix like this, antidepressants and/or psychotherapy may be more effective than HRT.

TIP: Depression is often worst first thing in the morning. It can be hard to get going and the temptation might be to stay in bed. Don't. Get up gently, and do something you can focus on as best you can, that isn't too taxing. If you feel you've accomplished something, it will help lift your mood. Reward yourself for this achievement and then, if you feel up to it, try undertaking another small task. Always stop before you get exhausted and remember to be kind to yourself throughout the day.

Q&A

Sarah: So if low mood is common at this time, would you say the menopause actually causes anxiety and depression?

Patrick: I think it's tricky to separate complex processes that may be happening at the same time; it's better to look at the whole person and take a holistic approach. I don't feel anxiety and depression and the menopause are inextricably linked, so that if you're perimenopausal, then anxiety and/or depression are inevitable. Nor do I think that they are separate entities. Instead I see anxiety or depression in the perimenopause as a reflection of the whole woman and what's going on in her life.

   If we look at the bigger picture, she'll be experiencing hormonal changes at what is often an emotionally-charged time. She may be sensing sorrow at the loss of her fertility and youth, perhaps worrying about her looks (often this is fuelled by newspapers, social media and peer opinion) and starting to fear old age. She is probably more conscious of her own mortality than she was, and may be feeling the loss of her mothering role in the family if her children are leaving home. Or she might be living with teenagers, who can be testing even when we're at the top of our game, or managing a parent whose failing memory is both upsetting and exasperating. This is a potent collection of triggers – and sometimes there may be a background of anxiety and/or depression as well – so frankly, if a woman in this situation *weren't* somewhat anxious or depressed, I'd be surprised! But that is not the same as saying that the menopause causes anxiety and/or depression. Not every menopausal woman is bound to experience anxiety or depression, or even if they do that they don't necessarily all need medical help. Everyone experiences mood changes – even my dog and your cat.

I find it's more helpful to establish when anxiety or depression become a problem, or, as I think of it, pathological. That is, causing illness. If anxiety or depression get to a level that your day-to-day functioning is compromised, when things we take for granted like getting up, commuting, going out, taking care of yourself (eating/washing/sleeping) and self-worth become impossible, then help is needed. Ideally, *before* it gets that bad. And if your menopausal symptoms are compounding this, then we need to address both problems, but not separately, because you are one person. I'd advise you to:

- Make a list of the concerns and worries you feel are effecting your health and wellbeing
- Look at your list and order the items according to how much they worry you
- Then talk through the list, one item at a time, with a loved one, your partner, someone in your family, a friend, or even – dare I say it – your doctor

Having someone to listen can ease the lid off the pressure cooker. Sometimes a solution is simple, but most of us benefit from multiple levels of support and care. That support might come from family and/or friends, it might be psychologically therapeutic, it may be medicinal, or it might be a combination of these. And if you feel you can't talk to anyone you know, then, if you're desperate, **phone the Samaritans on 08457 90 90 90** in the UK. They are excellent at listening in a non-judgemental way.

If you're suffering from depression or very low mood, you might like to read *Making Peace with Depression* – you'll find details at the back of this book. You could also consider joining the *Making Friends with Anxiety & Depression* support group on Facebook which I mentioned earlier

If you have been very down for a while, especially if you are having thoughts of self harming, **it's important you ask for help.** There's no shame in admitting you are depressed; it's not your *fault*. It's also possible to get better, although if you're in this frame of mind it can be hard to see the light at the end of the tunnel. As Patrick says, talk to someone you're close to about how you're feeling, and make a time to see your GP to discuss the options.

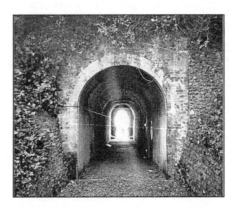

2.4 'Oh my God, I want to kill someone!' – Anger

'The female of the species is much deadlier than the male.'

Rudyard Kipling

Some women find that during the menopausal years their levels of tolerance seem to vanish. This causes them to explode, fast and with no warning. **BOOM!** Like a bomb going off, their rage is extreme and hurts others, and it often triggers regret. If you're finding you're much more hot-tempered and irritable than you used to be, it can be very unsettling.

As we've mentioned, middle age is a time of lots of life changes aside from the menopause, many of which can be stressful. **Throw in increased tiredness as a result of insomnia (a common effect of menopause which we'll come onto), raised levels of adrenaline and reduced progesterone and perhaps it's not *so* surprising we end up behaving as if we're waging war on the world after all.** It's rare for fury to come *completely* out of the blue, so whilst it may seem that your emotions are out of control when you explode, if you examine what triggered you in its totality you may well find there were several contributing factors – including hormonal change.

Clinician Marcy Holmes explains that if you previously had a tendency to experience premenstrual symptoms, the more extreme hormone fluctuations of perimenopause can exaggerate your symptoms tenfold. **The complicated and delicate balance of hormones can get out of kilter in perimenopause, which can impact the feel-good chemistry of the brain and cause extreme emotions,** including rage.

'It was difficult to deal with all the anger I had, especially as I had no idea what it was about. It was lucky that I was living in the country, and being in the middle of nowhere helped that process. I could stomp up a hill and scream and rant and roar. But meeting new people was hard, because I didn't know who this angry person was.' **Holly, 54**

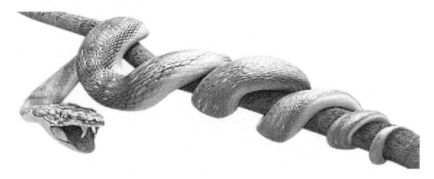

2.5 Taking care of our own mental health

In the summary, NICE guidelines recommend self-help groups, psychotherapy, counselling or antidepressants for psychological symptoms of menopause, plus HRT for anxiety. It's important to remember that all these are suggestions and which, if any, is right for you depends upon your preference. But before resorting to medication, why not try a natural and nutritional approach? The key is promoting balance again, says Holmes. She has worked closely with women of all ages and the common theme she's observed is that sugar, caffeine, alcohol and stress will exaggerate any hormonal symptoms. Unstable blood sugar and an over-activated stress response – on top of hormone fluctuations – create a perfect storm for emotional outbursts and perimenopausal rage. She urges that we try to curb these dietary triggers and pay more attention to what we put into our bodies, so that our brains can cope better with the hormone changes of perimenopause.

Looking after our minds involves caring for our bodies, and given this complex state of physiological affairs, it stands to reason that throughout the perimenopause balancing your hormones, addressing possible thyroid issues, eating a diet balanced with protein, fat, and complex carbohydrates, along with moderate daily exercise are particularly helpful. **Often our moods can be managed through lifestyle changes, such as learning ways to relax and reduce stress**.

- Exercise and eat healthily
- Find a self-calming skill to practise, such as yoga, meditation, or rhythmic breathing

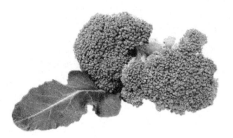

- Avoid tranquilizers and alcohol
- Engage in a creative outlet that fosters a sense of achievement – learn to play an instrument, take up painting, sewing or carpentry – what appeals to you?
- Nurture your friendships
- Stay connected with your family and community
- And, if you can, remember to laugh – or at least smile – at yourself and life in general

One of the main psychological issues connected to the menopause is that there is a danger of getting lost in emotions and

making judgments or decisions about your life based on feelings that are linked to your hormones changing. This is where some of the practices I learned when struggling to manage my anxiety are useful. One trick is to **try not to 'catastrophize'**, i.e. decide in advance that catastrophe is inevitable.

TIP: 'When you wake up tomorrow, rather than think: "I'm going to have an anxious day and feel rubbish", you could venture to consider: "Today might be OK after all". Sometimes it seems like there's no alternative, but if you give it a go you might be surprised to discover there often is.' **Sarah Rayner, Making Friends with Anxiety**

Another useful exercise is to **try and get some distance from your emotions.** Often easier said than done, but it can be helpful to see yourself as your own best friend, advising yourself as she or he would do. Should your mind start to chatter or whirl, see your thoughts as mental events that come and go, like clouds across a sky. Gently acknowledge those thoughts, then imagine watching them float away.

According to **Carol S. Parsons,** we need to develop a part of ourselves that can stand back and watch with independent judgement. She explains in her book *Red Moon Passage* how we can benefit from taking our experiences less personally and seeing them in a broader context, as part of a process which all women on the planet go through. If we can differentiate between ourselves and our emotions, then it's less likely we'll be controlled by our feelings. It's a lot like puberty, with one difference – we are wiser, and we can put this wisdom to good use by learning from feelings but not allowing them to take us over. Nonetheless Parsons believes that this doesn't mean blocking or repressing emotions, or even transcending them, but still having them fully.

If, after doing your best to live in a way that cares for your mind and body, you're *still* struggling emotionally, it's probably time to consult your doctor. The issue is not that you *should* be able to deal with everything life throws at you, or that 'other women' seem to manage better. **What matters is whether you are coping or not coping,** as Patrick has said. **If you're *not* coping, make that call.**

'It's shockingly underrated how awful – truly unwell – the menopause can make you feel. The effect on mood is hideously underestimated. The sad thing is that women can feel like this for two or three years before it gets so unbearable that they approach their doctor. I had the first signs of perimenopause at 42, but didn't go to my doctor until I was 45. The difference a good (or bad) GP can make is so crucial – I was lucky, mine didn't mess around trying to measure hormones in a non-existent cycle – he added symptoms to age (even though I was relatively young) and said, "So – here are your options." Also, don't base your treatment decisions on what the tabloid media say. Read books on the subject; for me knowing what to expect, knowing it is all normal (albeit hell!) gave me a sense of control, so in the lows I see it as just a symptom and think of it like a very annoying cold!' **Nic, 48**

It's also important to **remember that whilst it can seem as if it's lasting for a lifetime, the menopause is not forever**. Once postmenopause is reached, the turbulence of hormone imbalance and the symptoms it causes will be over. Until that time, brace yourselves, dear readers, and be gentle with your body and soul.

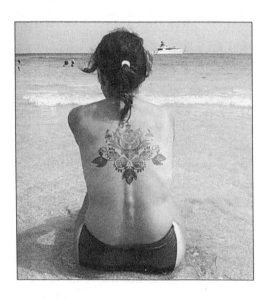

3.   'N' is for Nighttime

The menopause can have a significant impact on us at night. Let's find out why.

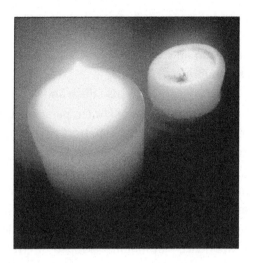

3.1 Hot flushes and night sweats

'What dreadful hot weather we have! It keeps me in a perpetual state of inelegance.'

Jane Austen, excerpt from a letter, **September 18 1796**

Hot flushes and night sweats (also called 'vasomotor symptoms') are the most commonly reported symptoms of menopause, with a significant proportion of those being severely affected.

It's perhaps surprising, given their prevalence and how uncomfortable they can make us feel, that the cause of hot flushes is yet to be established with 100% certainty. Doctors used to believe that they were caused purely by falling oestrogen, but practitioners such as Ray Peat have argued that it suited both medics and the industry that grew up around oestrogen-based HRT not to question this assumption too deeply. Whether or not this is true, the picture does seem more complicated than that, and recent research on animals suggests the brain plays a vital part. Falling oestrogen has been mooted as affecting the hypothalamus, a deep brain structure that, in part, helps regulate body temperature. It's now proposed that the hypothalamus is responsible for the release neurotransmitters that dilate peripheral arteries resulting in flushing but more research is needed to verify this, so let's focus instead on the pressing issues: how hot flushes and night sweats affect us, and what we can do when they happen.

- Hot flushes commonly affect the face, head, neck and chest, and last for a few minutes.
- As well as sweating, you may also flush and become red.
- Hot flushes tend to raise your skin temperature, but at the same time your internal temperature can drop.
- Depending on the severity of the hot flush, you may get a headache or feel weak and dizzy.
- Hot sweats are more common in the evening and, as you might expect, during hot weather.
- Your heart rate and blood flow also increase, which is why you may also experience palpitations (skipped or erratic heart beats) along with the hot flush or night sweat.
- As your body toils to correct the imbalance, you can become chilled and shivery.
- At night this chain reaction can make you sweat heavily and awaken you from sleep.
- Night sweats can last anything from one minute up to one hour, and can occur every hour or just a couple of times a week.

*'For me, the sensation of a hot flush is totally different to how I feel when I get overheated from being in a warm environment or from physical exertion. It's a **bit** like when you realize with a shock that something has gone horribly wrong and you get a sudden flash of heat through your whole body. But that tends to feel like a rush of blood, whereas a hot flush is more like having an internal furnace fired up. In my case, these flushes last for about ten seconds and, having looked in the mirror when they are happening, I know that my face and neck go blotchy and pink. Typically, these flushes are closely followed by a break-out of perspiration and it is this I find most troubling. I find it embarrassing to be talking to someone, perhaps in a shop or restaurant, and all of a sudden my face breaks out and is drenched in sweat.'* **Chloe, 48**

'I had about two years of intensive night sweats, where I would have liked to change my bedding every day. I didn't, because I have too much to do, but I longed to. It was awful. I was really glad I wasn't in a relationship as my sheets were soaked through.' **Holly, 54**

Relieving hot flushes

NICE recommend that lifestyle changes such as taking regular exercise, avoiding possible triggers for hot flushes and ensuring good sleep hygiene will help many women to manage their menopausal symptoms. Whilst HRT may be useful, the risks and benefits of treatment must be considered for each woman, they say, and for women who are unable or unwilling to use HRT, treatment options include fluoxetine, citalopram or venlafaxine.[1] These last three are more commonly prescribed as antidepressants – fluoxetine is also known by the brand name Prozac – so before turning to medication, it stands to reason that it's worth starting with changes to your home and wardrobe, diet and exercise regime.

- Wear lightweight clothes made of natural fibres such as cotton, wool and silk which allow your skin to breathe.
- Layering your clothes – particularly on your top half – means you can strip off more easily should you get hot.

'I highly recommend wearing layers. More than once I've found myself overheating horribly and because I've only been wearing one top, I couldn't strip off or I'd just be down to my bra!' **Juliet, 53**

- Dig out the gadgets you'd use in a heatwave – plug in the electric fan, switch on the air con – and invest in a mini handheld fan to carry in your handbag at all times, as well as a couple of cotton handkerchiefs.
- It might feel counter-intuitive when you're breaking out in hot sweats, but regular exercise can ease feeling over-warm. A study from Penn State University, US, found that exercise helped prevent the onset of hot flushes in the 24 hours after physical activity. It does this by:

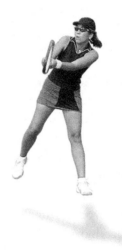

- Lowering the amount of Follicle Stimulating Hormone and Luteinizing Hormone (both of which stimulate your ovary to produce steroids).
- Raising your endorphin levels which will drop during a hot flush or night sweat.

- Research shows that overweight women who lose weight experience improvements in hot flushes. Specifically, for every 11 pounds lost, the likelihood of your hot flushes improving increases by one-third.

TIP: 'I wear less make-up than before – what's the point, when I'm going to be dabbing perspiration away and make-up with it? I wear looser and lighter clothes – just the thought of wearing a woolly polo neck makes me feel agitated – and try to avoid places that I know will be overbearingly warm and claustrophobic. But I always carry a small pack of wet wipes to freshen up with, just in case.' **Chloe, 48**

Relieving night sweats

- Keep your room as cool as you can – use a fan if need be

- Keep a cloth in a bucket of ice near your bed so you can cool yourself quickly
- Check your bedding isn't exacerbating your condition
- Progressive muscle relaxation, which involves tensing up each group of muscles then relaxing them can help reduce the frequency and severity of night sweats

TIP: *'After six months of awful night sweats, it dawned on me that our ancient duvet might not be helping. I swapped our 13.5 tog quilt, which was made of man-made fibre, for a 4.5 tog feather one. I also changed our polyester/cotton sheets to ones that are 100% Egyptian cotton. What a difference! Luckily my husband doesn't feel the cold, but if you've a partner who does, I'd suggest separate duvets – far better than tossing and turning all night.'* **Juliet, 53**

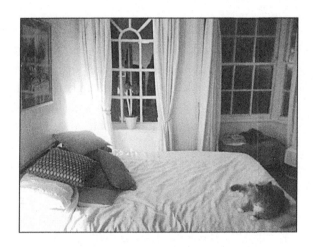

Some experts believe that hot flushes and night sweats deplete your body of vitamins B and C, magnesium and potassium, so it may be beneficial for you to increase your consumption of them. In addition, if you are carrying extra weight, slimming down may help.

During my research into night sweats, I came across this sentence online: *'Avoid or at least moderate possible triggers i.e. caffeine, alcohol, tobacco, spicy foods, hot drinks, white sugar, hot weather, hot baths, unexpressed anger and saunas/spa treatments.'* Perfectly valid point, but it made me smile; putting 'unexpressed anger' in the midst of a list which includes hot baths and spas seems to imply a powerful emotional response is as easily avoided as a sauna. Not in my experience it isn't – it can take months, possibly years, of therapy to become remotely *aware* of our unexpressed anger, never mind learning ways to avoid triggering it! Nevertheless, it's useful to be reminded that our minds and bodies are linked. Stress can exacerbate hot flushes – I can't count how often I've found myself burning up when I'm speaking in front of an audience or stuck in a traffic jam. Falling progesterone in perimenopause leaves us more vulnerable to stress and anxiety, as we saw in Chapter 2. This has led me to wonder if the sweating and flushing makes us feel increased anxiety because they resemble how we respond physically at anxious times. It then creates a vicious circle where the hot flush triggers anxiety, so hot flushes and night sweats intensify. It feels that way to me. Hopefully someone out there is doing the research!

Obviously it's good to minimize heated discussions (pardon the pun) and getting stuck in traffic jams if we can, but for me to suggest you 'avoid stress' would be glib. As if we can just turn off our lives like a bedside light – how I wish it were that simple! It can take time for the adrenaline to recede and to settle down again, and in this situation, I find it more helpful to bring my attention back to my breath.

TIP: Try slowing your breathing to five breaths per minute – four seconds breathing in; eight seconds breathing out.

The more we get upset and frustrated, the increasingly hot and bothered we're likely to become. Just as with anxiety, resistance is futile. Instead, **try and accept the physical sensations you are going through.** They're an outward sign of metamorphosis, says Susun S. Weed in her book *New Menopausal Years, The Wise Woman Way*, and we will be better off if we can relax and ride them like waves and honour them. So remind yourself that **neither anxiety nor hot flushes can harm you and aim to 'make friends' with the experience.**

'I have discovered that becoming anxious each time I wake with a night sweat is counter-productive to being able to fall back to sleep quickly, so I just try to

accept that doing the "hokey-cokey" all night with the sheets – one foot in, one foot out – is just the way I am currently!' **Chloe, 48**

Whilst hot flushes are extremely common, **no two women will have exactly the same internal thermostat.** I had hot flushes but not night sweats, and they only lasted about a year. Although they were inconvenient and uncomfortable, I didn't feel they were bad enough to consult my doctor, because I knew what they were. If you're finding night sweats are ruining your much-needed sleep, I imagine that's more distressing, and suggest you see your GP to discuss treatment. But before you go you might like to read up on HRT in Chapter 5 and alternative therapies in Chapter 6 so you've a broad understanding of the options.

3.2 Insomnia

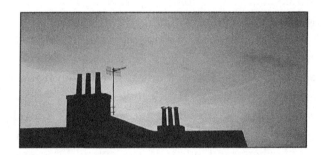

'A ruffled mind makes a restless pillow.' **Charlotte Brontë**

We've already discussed how waning levels of oestrogen and progesterone can increase the impact of adrenaline and make us more susceptible to anxiety, anger and hot flushes. **There's another stress hormone which can have a big impact on us as a result of falling reproductive hormones: cortisol.**

Cortisol, like adrenaline, is a powerful chemical released by the adrenal glands during the fight or flight response (see 2.2). But whereas adrenaline generally only lasts a relatively short time (which is why it's possible to ride out a hot flush or panic attack), cortisol helps us endure stress over a longer term. Adrenaline acts on the heart to increase heart rate, force muscle contraction and respiration; cortisol works on the liver and pancreas to increase glucose levels and make muscles easier to use. It also temporarily inhibits other systems of the body, including digestion, growth, reproduction and the immune system. Put very simply, adrenaline is what gives us the impetus to run from a lion; cortisol is what helps us cope with drought or famine.

Normally, cortisol is present in the body at higher levels in the morning and is at its lowest at night. When cortisol levels remain high, however, it can have a damaging effect on the body, just as adrenaline can. It's called a 'stress hormone' after all, and if we remain stressed for too long, it can interrupt sleep rhythms and prevent the restorative REM sleep cycle.

Sleep problems are not as common as hot flushes, yet they still affect 40-50% of women in menopausal transition, which, even if it improves in postmenopause, is an awful lot of us. Insomnia can be one of the most debilitating symptoms of perimenopause: in addition to making the other symptoms harder to bear, chronic insomnia has dangerous health implications: obesity, diabetes, hyper-tension, heart disease, depression, impaired immune function and, believe it or not, an increased risk for alcoholism. (Studies have shown that insomniacs often self-medicate with alcohol to induce sleep.)

As with low mood, **insomnia is likely to be exacerbated by other issues that are common at this time of life**. It's hard to relax if you're worried where your offspring has got to, for example, or if you're in the throes of moving to a smaller home because your kids have flown the nest. And sometimes it's hard to untangle whether we're worried and upset *because* we're not sleeping, or we're not sleeping because we're worried and upset, though in a way it doesn't really matter; what matters is to break the cycle, so we're sleeping better and maximizing our chances of feeling in a positive frame of mind.

So what should you do if menopause is preventing you from getting a good night's sleep? Let's start with an area that's relatively easy to tackle – creating habits and practices that are conducive to sleeping well on a regular basis. This is often referred to as 'sleep hygiene'. It's very important, says Joyce Walsleben, Head of

Behavioural Sleep Medicine at the NYU Center and Sleep Medicine Associates of NYC, because if we let poor sleep hygiene continue unchecked, we can 'learn' to have insomnia and adjust our life around it. The danger then is that even if our hormones *do* settle down, poor sleep hygiene has become established, which can prolong the impact of insomnia long after perimenopause.

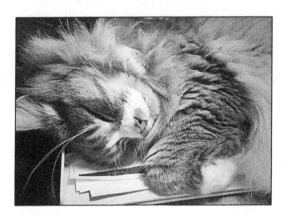

Improving sleep hygiene

In the day:

- Be consistent with your wake up time
- Avoid caffeine after 1pm or try decaffeinated drinks Fizzy drinks often contain caffeine, so check the contents
- Try committing to 30 minutes of exercise each day, as it's an excellent way to reduce stress and lower cortisol. Take it slow at first, and avoid exercising close to bedtime
- Avoid afternoon naps as they interrupt your sleep cycle
- A low-glycemic index diet (which includes complex carbohydrates) helps to control blood glucose levels, and as a result, has also been shown to reduce cortisol levels. Put simply: eat more fruit and vegetables and less fat
- Avoid eating a heavy meal after 8pm
- Don't drink alcohol or smoke

- Practice relaxation techniques such as yoga or meditation (see Chapter 6 for detail)

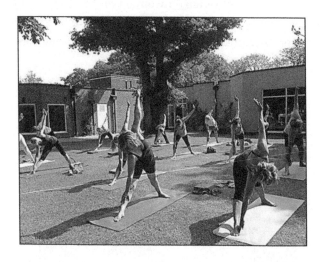

At night, build a tight sleep structure by paying attention to your environment:

- Give yourself time to fall asleep at night
- Don't use a laptop or mobile phone after 9pm – keep your mobile charging in another room if possible
- Make your room dark, quiet and safe

Before you get into bed, take a moment or two to pause and clear your head. Picture yourself throwing away thoughts that keep you awake. Imagine scrunching them up and putting them in the bin.

Further strategies to assist with sleep

Some find herbal remedies such as valerian and lavender beneficial. You might also like to try acupuncture or Shiatsu massage. Plus, if you have a Type-A, perfectionist personality (that'll be me then), now might be the time to see if you can learn to live with 'good enough', rather than striving to get an A* in everything. (There's more on this in *Making Friends with Anxiety*, so if it resonates you might benefit from taking a look.) After all, if your health depends on it, it's worth being less tough on yourself.

If, after a while, you are *still* finding symptoms of perimenopause are keeping you up or waking you up every night, make an appointment to see your doctor. He or she may suggest medication.

- HRT works by supplementing the oestrogen that is no longer being made by your body, boosting it to levels similar to before perimenopause. See Chapter 5 for more on the subject.
- A low-dose birth control pill can help stabilize milder fluctuations of oestrogen.
- Certain antidepressants can help stabilize sleep.

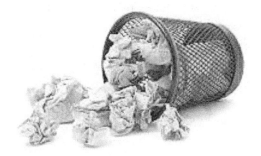

4.   'O' is for One-Size-Does-NOT-Fit-All

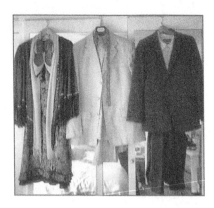

We've taken a look at the most common physical and psychological difficulties encountered during perimenopause and menopause, but what about those symptoms which are less common?

They can be equally uncomfortable and are sometimes more upsetting because we may not recognize that they're related to the menopause. They certainly deserve attention. Here are 11 examples:

- Itchy, crawling skin
- Tingling extremities
- Aching joints
- Forgetfulness
- Rapid heartbeat
- Dizziness or light-headedness
- Breast pain
- Bladder incontinence
- Increase in allergies
- Hair thinning
- Cracking/breaking fingernails

With all of these, as with other symptoms, **simple lifestyle changes can go a huge way to providing relief**. There's more on how to keep yourself physically and emotionally healthy as you age in Chapter 7, but Patrick's topline advice is that you aim to:

- Avoid caffeine and alcohol
- Sleep 7-8 hours per night
- Intake vitamins B, C, D, and E
- Practice breathing exercises
- Stay hydrated
- Eat a balanced diet
- Exercise regularly

You could even monitor your symptoms, and see if they improve.

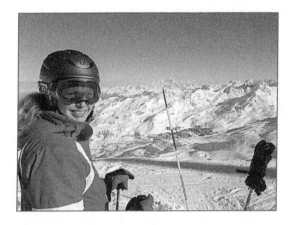

For some of us it's not so easy to get 7-8 hours' sleep every night, however – we've already discussed how insomnia is common in menopause. Equally, it's not always possible to find time to exercise as much as we'd like or to eat 100% healthily, especially if we're working and looking after a family, and for these reasons it's helpful to examine these specific symptoms in detail. That way, we'll understand what causes them and be better placed to manage as best we can within the confines of our own daily lives.

'I knew about hot flushes as they were the one symptom of menopause that gets talked about, so that wasn't what confused me. It was all the other stuff – the tiredness, the aches and pains, the emotional upheaval – that got me.'
Juliet, 53

4.1 Itchy, crawling skin

'I have felt a gradual slowing down over the past two years and several symptoms which I hadn't connected with menopause until joining the Facebook group, including very itchy skin.' **Chris, 49**

Itchy skin is thought to be caused by withdrawal of oestrogen. The changing ratio of hormones in your body does two things:

- It slows down your body's production of skin-smoothing collagen and oils
- It reduces your body's ability to retain moisture

Though ultimately harmless, having itchy skin can be maddening. I suffered from it in the latter stages of perimenopause myself and it was as if ants were crawling over my skin. It made concentrating on anything else very difficult!

Relieving skin complaints

- Use gentle soaps and bath products
- Avoid hot baths and showers, which dry skin out
- A diet rich in omega-3 fatty acids (found in fish like salmon and sardines, edamame beans, walnuts and many kinds of plant oil) helps keep skin healthy

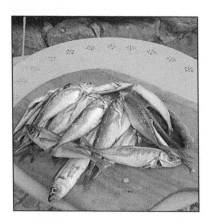

- Moisturise your skin regularly. I'd recommend a non-scented dermatological emollient (such as Cetraben, E45, Oilatum or Diprobase). Please be aware that these creams are flammable and can be dangerous should they get embedded in clothing.

4.2 Tingling extremities

Have you noticed a pins-and-needles sensation in your hands and feet becoming more frequent? Are you experiencing sensations of numbness, tingling, creeping and pain?

It's important to seek prompt medical evaluation for any persistent tingling in your extremities, as it can be a sign of another underlying health condition such as diabetes. What you may not know is that **pins and needles (known as 'paraesthesis') can also be a symptom of menopause.** Fluctuating hormones have a complex effect on the central nervous system and this can extend to your hands and feet. In particular a lack of oestrogen can cause the skin to become thinner and less elastic leading to tingling in the extremities and limbs.

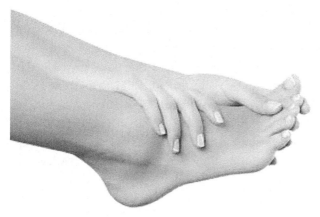

Relief for tingling extremities

In most cases, tingling extremities are simply a nuisance causing mild pain, numbness and burning. However, sometimes they can lead to a temporary inability to grip with the fingers and carry out delicate movements and some women can lose their balance while walking, due to numbness in their toes. If you're suffering badly, regular exercise can help, so try a combination of daily aerobic activity such as swimming, jogging at a light pace and walking, together with relaxation such as yoga, breathing exercises and visualization.

Occasionally tingling extremities can arise as a consequence of anxiety or accompany other menopausal symptoms such as joint pain. In these instances treatment of one symptom may alleviate the other, but if you're at all worried please see your doctor.

4.3 Aching joints

'If I had known I was going to live this long, I would have taken better care of myself.' **Mae West**

Last summer, I noticed my knees felt very stiff when I went up and down stairs. Am I destined to feel this creaky for the rest of my days? I thought to myself. Dear me, what on earth will I be like in ten years' time?

But feeling less flexible is not always a sign of worse joint problems to come as you age. Dr Rod Hughes, consultant rheumatologist at St Peter's Hospital, Chertsey, Surrey explains, 'Perimenopausal women can also get a lot of hip pain, in particular over the outside of the hips. These pains are not, in fact, anything to do with the hip joints, which still move freely, but are the result of tenderness in tissues between muscles.' He says that this **stiffness and inflammation in the soft tissues around the joints is caused by a drop in oestrogen**. Once we're through the menopause, our bodies can regain flexibility.

Relief for aching joints

- Stretching exercises such as yoga, pilates and swimming are particularly good for aching joints.
- Weight training can also help to build more muscle.

74

- It may be worth looking closely at what you eat, and experimenting with an 'anti-inflammatory diet'. This sounds complex, but much of it is common sense, really:
  - Aim for variety
  - Include as much fresh food as possible
  - Minimise your consumption of processed foods and fast food
  - Ensure your plate is about 2/3 vegetables
  - With the remaining 1/3, explore a variety of foods. From oily fish to pulses – whatever takes your fancy
  - Try to include carbohydrates, fat and protein at each meal
  - Eat fruit instead of crisps or other snacks

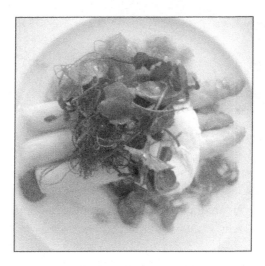

- If that sounds doable, you might like to go a step further. See if you can implement the following too:
  - The distribution of calories you take in should be 40-50% from carbohydrates, 30% from fat, and 20-30% from protein
  - Reduce your consumption of foods made with wheat flour and sugar, especially bread and most packaged snack foods (including crisps)
  - Eat more whole grains such as brown rice and bulgar wheat, in which the grain is intact. (Please note: if you have Coeliac Disease, this is not advisable)

- Eat more beans, winter squash and sweet potatoes
- Cook pasta 'al dente' and eat it in moderation

If you do change your diet, why not share your findings in the *Making Friends with the Menopause* Facebook group? I'm sure other members will be interested to hear.

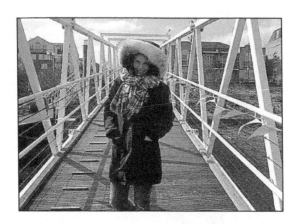

4.4 Forgetfulness

Another effect of menopause that can cause alarm is forgetfulness. It's all too easy to convince ourselves we're on a slippery slope to dementia, and get anxious we'll never remember another person's name again, whereas it may well be your hormones making mischief with your mind.

Research has shown that **changes in cognitive brain function – including how we remember things – can be a symptom of menopause**. Oestrogen has a role to play in our brains: it elevates levels of neurotransmitters such as serotonin, promotes neuron growth and the formation of synapses, acts as an antioxidant and has a regulatory effect on messenger systems. As it drops, so we become subject to memory loss, but it doesn't mean that our ability to remember will necessarily continue to get worse.

Tackling memory loss

Struggling with forgetfulness? Here are some ways to care of yourself:

- Regular exercise will increase the heart rate and flow of oxygenated blood. It will also release endorphins and improve sleep, which can help the brain.

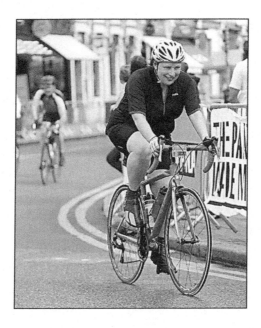

- Drink up to 2-3 litres of water a day – water hydrates the body and brain, and is vital for both to function well.
- Mind games such as Sudoku and crosswords keep your brain active.
- Learning a new skill will stimulate your brain to make new connections.
- Socialisation is important too – don't cut off your friends and family.
- Certain foods such as oily fish, soy products, fruit and vegetables have been shown to improve mental function, so including these in your diet may help with your memory lapses.
- Getting a good amount of sleep has been proven to increase mental function and concentration. Whereas if you spend your waking hours tired, your ability to remember information will reduce.

- If you begin to panic when your brain denies you information, this will only make the situation worse, so it's important to try to find ways to relax, which we'll explore more presently.

4.5 Heart palpitations and feeling giddy

It can be frightening to sense your heart pounding, fluttering or beating irregularly, even if it's just for a few seconds. However, palpitations are not usually a sign of a problem with your heart – often they are stress-related, which is why people with high levels of anxiety are susceptible. **We've already seen how anxiety can increase in the run up to menopause, and the same is true of heart palpitations.** They can also be connected to consumption of alcohol or tobacco, as can feeling giddy, and during menopause both palpitations and giddiness can be compounded by oestrogen withdrawal. Nonetheless if you experience either it's important that you get checked out by your GP, especially if your palpitations are accompanied by a feeling of tightness in your chest.

Managing palpitations and dizziness

I hope you don't need this little book to point out that smoking is unwise, but what you may not know is that women who smoke typically have an earlier menopause than non-smokers, and suffer more greatly with symptoms. The same is true of alcohol and caffeine, and together these have a cumulative effect. Add stress and/or being overweight into the mix, and you're increasing the likelihood of palpitations and dizziness making your journey through menopause considerably more difficult, which is why it's worth making every effort to implement some of the lifestyle changes mentioned throughout this book.

4.6 Breast pain in one or both breasts

Breast pain, soreness or tenderness in one or both breasts is symptomatic of hormonal changes, and often precedes or accompanies menstruation, and can also occur during pregnancy,

post-partum and menopause. The specific imbalance of hormones that causes breast pain is unique to each individual, so sensitivity might occur at different times or at different intensities in any one of us.

Other breast pain triggers include caffeine, poor diet and breast size. While discomfort during menopause is very rarely a sign of cancer, it is never a bad idea to speak with a doctor. It's also important to have your breasts examined regularly.

Self-care for breast pain

- Go for a walk for half an hour each day
- Wear a supportive bra while exercising, even sleeping
- Use towel-wrapped ice packs to ease pain
- Experiment with visualization and breathing techniques
- Increase dietary fibre (good sources include beans, raspberries and avocado)
- Look for natural diuretics - fennel, celery and cucumber
- Reduce salt intake to 6g (a teaspoon) a day

4.7 Loss of bladder control

Bladder incontinence is not an inevitable consequence of the menopause. Although **some experts believe that it is connected to lowering oestrogen levels which cause the pelvic floor muscles to lose strength, research shows other causes are more likely**. Worsening anxiety, a high baseline BMI and weight gain (which often arise at this time of life too) can also cause urinary incontinence. All these affect the urethra, the tube that passes urine from the bladder out of the body and, combined with weakened pelvic floor muscles, common in women in midlife, can lead to leakage.

Relief for urinary incontinence

- Using exercises to strengthen pelvic floor muscles (these are the muscles you use to stop urinating mid-stream) can make a big difference. Contracting and relaxing them is the key – try these on patient.co.uk to start off with.

- Drinks with caffeine or alcohol fill the bladder more quickly (they have a diuretic action) so try to cut back.
- Gradually retrain your bladder to hold more urine by only urinating at certain, pre-planned times of the day.
- Losing weight reduces the pressure on your bladder and muscles.

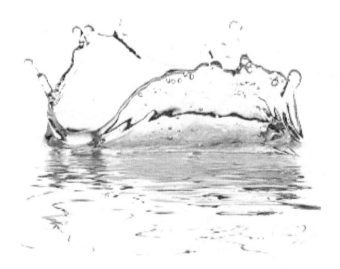

4.8 An increase in allergies

You've doubtless come across hay fever and asthma, as well as allergies to house dust, bee stings, nuts and certain medications. Put simply, an allergy is the result of the immune system overreacting to a foreign substance. In an attempt to protect the body, an allergic person produces the antibody, immunoglobulin E. We all generate this antibody, but in the allergic person it is produced in abnormal amounts.

Although some people live with allergies from childhood, they often develop when the body is under stress, and the significant hormonal shifts of puberty, menstruation, pregnancy and menopause can exacerbate allergic reactions. **Sometimes allergies worsen during** menopause, sometimes new allergies arise, and some women see an increase in respiratory symptoms associated with asthma.

Treatment

Over-the-counter and prescribed medication can bring relief but may make you drowsy, so it pays to know your triggers and take preventative measures. It's worth noting that a survey by the National Pollen and Aerobiology Research Unit of more than 2,000 people found that stress and exercise can have a major impact on allergies like hay fever. When stress levels drop, symptoms lessen; equally, those who exercise most have the mildest symptoms. If your allergies have got worse during the menopause, you might like to consider activities such as tai chi, yoga and meditation to help relax the mind and body.

'For me, joint and connective tissue pains have been the most unpleasant and least expected side effects of the menopause. But the most curious has to be the onset and exacerbation of allergies – hay fever is one thing, but cherries?'
Bernadette, 52

4.9 Thinning hair

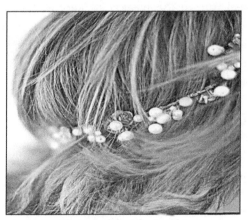

Photograph by John Knight

Most people consider hair loss to be a man's problem, so if you notice your brush has more hair in it, this can be quite a shock. Yet **thinning**

81

of the hair can occur as a result of the hormonal changes we go through in menopause. Women's menopausal hair loss tends to be more diffuse and spread evenly throughout the scalp, leading to overall thinning as opposed to actual baldness. Nonetheless, it can contribute to poor self-esteem so if you are very distressed, you might like to discuss the issue with your GP as HRT can help. If you have bald spots, it is more likely to be alopecia, which is not menopause-related, and you should consult your doctor.

4.10 Brittle nails

While many other symptoms of perimenopause and menopause can have a serious effect on your life, brittle nails may not. However, they too can knock your self-esteem and make you self-conscious about your appearance, which can then have a wider impact on your relationships.

Each fingernail is made of keratin, which is formed by cells located at the base of the nail bed. When women are healthy and their hormones are properly balanced, these cells function properly, and keratin is strong and sturdy. **Once we reach menopause, the accompanying hormonal imbalances can lead to brittle nails that tear, split or peel due to the weakened keratin layer.** The result is primarily cosmetic, but in some cases, anaemia, poor circulation or low thyroid functioning can contribute to brittle nails, so if you're feeling unwell and suspect you may have another condition, it's worth going to see your doctor.

Treatment for thinning hair and brittle nails

In most cases, brittle nails and thinning hair are simply caused by the hormonal changes of menopause. Good nutrition with the right balance of nutrients, including protein, calcium, iron, vitamin C, fat and folic acid are essential for a healthy head of hair and strong nails, while regular exercise can stimulate circulation and improve overall health. Again, reducing stress by practising meditation or trying relaxing forms of exercise such as yoga and pilates can be helpful.

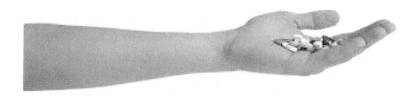

4.11 Further unusual menopausal symptoms

If you are experiencing a symptom not listed here, it *doesn't* mean it isn't related to the menopause. It may be we didn't have room in this book. If you've noticed your body changing and you're wondering if it could be connected to hormonal change, the website **34-menopause-symptoms.com** may help.

'I have had to accept that I'm very tired. My acupuncturist said, "It's the most underrated symptom of the menopause, and you have to take notice of it, and look after it. You have to rest". That was unexpected. I remember my mother lying down in the afternoon when I was a teenager, and she was going through the menopause, but I never thought I'd be doing that.' **Holly, 54**

4.12 Communicating with your doctor

After learning that a symptom that you didn't know was related to the menopause is connected to your changing hormones, many women are relieved to learn that we do not have some dreaded disease. **Aside from accessing treatment, we appreciate being in the know and learning that we are not imagining things.** It empowers us to discover that our experiences are natural and part of being women.

This was certainly true for me when I found out increased anxiety is something others sometimes experience at this time in their lives: I went from being confused and scared to comforted, knowing I wasn't alone. However, as I've mentioned in Chapter 2, I didn't find it easy to get an expert to see things the same way, and unfortunately, other women report similar difficulties.

Take 51-year-old Janet, for example. 'Two years ago I started to get shooting pains in my neck, which spread to both shoulders and down my limbs. I felt spasms in my back and legs the whole time and I was in constant pain. I went from being a fit, flexible 49-year-old to a

50-year-old who could barely move. I could never get comfortable, and nothing seemed to help. I went to my doctor, and was prescribed strong painkillers, but they barely took the edge off the agony. He sent me for a brain scan which revealed nothing, and a chiropractor tried everything he could, but again, no joy. Eventually I looked on a forum online, where I discovered that nerve and joint pain is sometimes linked to menopause.'

Janet read another woman's similar story, then another and another, and learned (as we touched on earlier in this chapter) that **in a small percentage of women oestrogen fluctuations can have an impact on the soft tissue around the joints, which then manifests itself as abnormally severe pain and menopausal arthritis.** Like other conditions described in this chapter, it is not an 'obvious' symptom of perimenopause.

'So I marched straight back to my GP and told him that I thought my joint pain was related to my being menopausal,' Janet says. 'He'd not heard of this before, but he agreed to my trying HRT for a month. Honestly, the difference was incredible. I started the HRT, within a month I felt so much better and now, three months later, I'm back to my old self.'

Whilst Patrick and I would not recommend that you try to diagnose yourself online as it can work the other way and make us worry about diseases we *don't* have, Janet's story does highlight some important issues.

- **Every woman's experience of the menopause is unique**
- Whilst hot flushes and irregular periods are very common, **you may experience other, less common effects of the menopause**
- **Sometimes you have to push for an effective diagnosis**
- No matter what other people say – including me and Patrick – **you're the one inhabiting your own skin, and only *you* know what that feels like**

All this said, it's also worth reminding ourselves that **GPs are only human**. Your doctor may not – indeed *cannot* – know every symptom of every condition known to man and woman. Remember that they have to deal with all sorts of diseases and conditions, and are required to know about a vast range of possibilities in terms of diagnosis. In any one day they are likely to have to see babies and OAPs, patients with terminal cancer and patients with common colds. GPs also have individual strengths and weaknesses, like the rest of us, and, although as patients we're often unaware of this, some are more interested in particular areas of healthcare than others.

How to get the most from a consultation with your GP

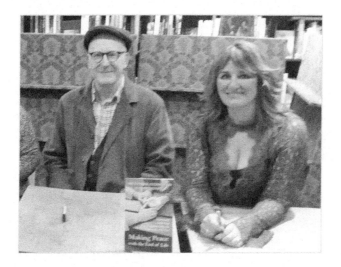

'Togetherness is strength.' **John-Bertrand Aristide**

<u>Q&A</u>

Sarah: Have you any tips on how to get the best from your GP? Over the years I've had many different doctors, some good, some bad. When I had really awful anxiety, my GP was brilliant. But last year I saw another doctor as mine was unavailable and he just wouldn't listen. I came away feeling worse than before I went. How can I help my doctor help me?

Patrick: To have some effect on this disparity, it may be worth arming yourself for the consultation beforehand. Bear in mind your GP has 10 minutes to go through your concerns, examine you as necessary, formulate a plan you're both happy with, and then write it up. Plus, as you say, your doctor is human and will be affected by the stories they hear every 10 minutes, and it's good to remember that. I'd suggest that the following may help you plan for an optimal consultation:

1. See the right doctor – do you want a male or female? Ask. Do you not want a specific doctor because of previous problems? Tell the receptionist. It may mean you have to wait a little longer to see the doctor of your choice, but usually menopausal symptoms are not emergencies and the symptoms have been there for some time.

2. Make a list. You're here about your menopausal symptoms and worries. So write them down – all of them, but stick to the subject. If you start asking about a second issue you're going to flummox the GP who has 10 minutes to try to support you with a highly complex problem and you're not going to get the focus you need. (Have I said 10 minutes enough times?) Make another appointment if you have a second, unrelated problem.

3. Tell the GP what you think may be going on. It helps establish your concerns around your symptoms and you can also be reassured if you are worried about something unnecessarily. However, if you think you may have something more serious then tell the doctor too. e.g. family histories of diseases – these vital clues help to build a picture.

4. Allow the GP to ask you questions, even if they seem irrelevant. They are sifting through information to make sure nothing untoward is going on. If there is a history of cancer or blood clots in your family your GP needs to know this as it affects HRT prescribing. Smoking and alcohol information are needed – don't be upset, it's not a judgement or being nosey – we need this to help find the safest way forward.

5. Ask your GP what the options are. It may be doing nothing. It may be taking blood tests. It may be medication. It may be counselling. What do you expect to happen? Tell them what you are expecting. If our GP doesn't know what you're hoping for then they may assume other ways forward.

6. Make a follow up appointment, if needs be, to see how the changes have gone. Changes take time – so wait at least 2-3 weeks before checking in.

If you feel you didn't connect with your GP, don't get angry. It may have been the consultation before yours that involved something so upsetting that they couldn't concentrate. It may be that they should retire! Make an appointment with another doctor until you find the one who suits you. Though be warned: it may not be the one who gives you lots and lots of time as they may be dithering around decisions. Remember, your doctor is there to support you. They can't fix your life, but most GPs do aim to listen to your worries and provide guidance to the best of their abilities.

Don't just *assume* that your symptoms are due to menopause, they may not be. Many of the symptoms mentioned are indicators of other conditions too – pins and needles can be a sign of diabetes for instance, and feeling giddy can be caused by low blood pressure. Your doctor may want to rule these out first, so try to keep an open mind and be kind to yourself *and* your GP. In my experience, a little empathy in everyday interactions often goes a long way.

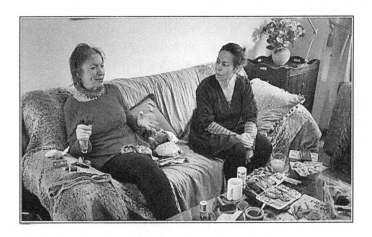

If, after all this, you *still* feel your GP is not diagnosing you accurately, you are entitled to ask for a second opinion. Alternatively,

you might like to push for a referral. Search for a specialist who is local to you on **menopausematters.co.uk**, a very useful website.

TIP: Sometimes it's worth having a discreet word with the receptionist at your surgery to find which doctor they believe is best equipped to help you manage your menopausal symptoms. Choose the time to mention this carefully (avoid Monday morning for instance, when you might get short shrift) and ask him or her for advice.

'I don't think it's fair to expect our GPs to be able to fine-tune what HRT we need – they're not specialists and only have ten minutes per appointment. If, like me, you're a complicated case – though really, who isn't, when it comes down to it? – I'd recommend that you ask for a referral to a gynaecologist or endocrinologist. Personally, I'd like to see more referrals given by GPs.' **Stella, 58**

'Fortunately, the majority of menopausal symptoms will get better after your body has adapted to the new hormone levels,' **says Patrick. 'Hot flushes will ease, your skin will stop itching, your joint flexibility will return and your memory will improve again. But I appreciate it's impossible to know exactly how long these symptoms will last as each woman is different and if you're finding them very distressing, I'd say it's worth considering HRT to replace the oestrogen that your ovaries are no longer producing. HRT doesn't suit everyone, and it has its drawbacks, but for some women it's transformative, enabling to them to live life to the full again, rather than longing for the menopause to be over.'**

Which leads, very neatly, to our next chapter.

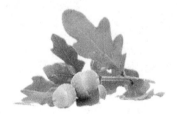

5. 'P' is for Pressing 'Pause' – the pros and cons of HRT

Traditionally, medical treatment for menopause has tended to revolve around Hormone Replacement Therapy (HRT), which can help alleviate many of the symptoms associated with falling levels of oestrogen. What are the pitfalls, if any?

'Having HRT was like pressing a "pause" button on the changes my body was going through. I felt like I'd been fast-forwarding into old age, becoming this creaky old woman, and suddenly it was like I'd stopped the clock, even rewound it a couple of years, back to when I was 49.' **Janet, 51**

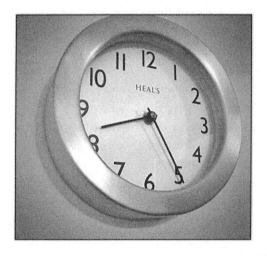

We've seen that in the run-up to our final period and during menopause, declining reproductive hormones can have a major impact on our physical and mental health. But it can be hard to work out if HRT is the way forward, especially when there are different kinds available, and you might have heard conflicting reports about the risks. We can't promise to resolve every single issue concerning HRT, but let's try to unravel some of the confusion.

5.1 What is HRT?

We've discussed how fluctuating oestrogen, in particular, can trigger different responses in each of us. Some women experience hot flushes, some suffer from joint aches and pins and needles, others are prone to mood swings and so on. According to **www.patient.co.uk** around 80% of women are impacted by declining hormones in some way, so it makes sense that HRT aims to replace oestrogen and counteract the consequences of this reduction in oestrogen.

Nonetheless **HRT shouldn't be viewed as one intervention with set risks and side effects.** The duration, severity and impact of the perimenopause and menopause vary hugely between women, and the effects vary from month to month for any one individual. Just as there's no 'one-size-fits-all' experience of menopausal symptoms, there's no 'one-size-fits-all' response in terms of hormone replacement either. Oestrogen comes in different forms and can be taken as a daily tablet, twice weekly or weekly patch, or as a gel applied daily.

In addition, oestrogen cannot be taken on its own unless you have had a hysterectomy as it can cause thickening of the womb lining, increasing the risk of endometrial cancer. Therefore, if you still have your womb, most doctors now recommend taking progestogen (the name for synthetically-produced progesterone) along with oestrogen, because progestogen can protect the womb lining. Progestogen can be taken in tablet or patch form and is available in some preparations combined with oestrogen. Another way of taking progestogen is via the Mirena intrauterine system which releases it directly into the cavity of the womb. There's more on the different types of HRT at the end of this chapter.

5.2 What are the benefits of HRT?

For women who experience an early or premature menopause, the benefits of HRT can be considerable. Most women in this situation are advised to take HRT until their early 50s, i.e. the average age of the menopause, and it can help restore a sense of physical and mental wellbeing.

Regardless of the age we go through the menopause, oestrogen reduction can still have a major impact on our quality of life, so it's little surprise **symptom control is by far the most common reason for taking HRT.**

'I had keyhole surgery on my fibroids in my late forties, and two weeks after the op I started to have really bad hot flushes, especially at night. I went to my GP as I was hardly sleeping and he prescribed HRT meds and within two days I felt fine again. I am still on the tablets, and although I put on half a stone in weight I am really happy with the hormone replacement. I'm in a relationship with another woman, and my sexual appetite has not changed with all of this. My mother had the same symptoms and was on HRT meds for 20 years – she says it helped her keep her bones strong and the hot flushes at bay. So I guess I am following her lead, though I don't intend to stay on HRT as long as she did.' **Carol, 49**

If you suffer from hot flushes, night sweats or insomnia, mood swings, or many of more unusual other symptoms we looked at in Chapter 4, the odds are very high that HRT will provide relief. **Research has shown that HRT can reduce symptoms like these by as much as 80%.** This in turn can have a positive effect on family life, relationships and work.

In addition, research has shown that HRT can reduce the risk of various diseases and conditions associated with ageing if started within a few years of your periods stopping.

'I have a longstanding history of anxiety and depression which had been well controlled for 20 years with antidepressants. I went to my doctor when I was 52 complaining of a sudden and dramatic return of my anxiety symptoms. (I had been having periods about once every four months and was about to have my last period, although of course at the time I didn't know that.) I asked if the symptoms could be connected to my menopause and was told no, and I was also told that HRT is not given to women of my age – only to younger women who are at risk of bone problems. I then spent two years trying to control dreadful anxiety and depression for which antidepressants only partly worked (I even lost my job during this period due to having too much time off work and was dismissed on health grounds).

When the recent NICE guidelines made the news, I went to see a private doctor through my work and was immediately put on an HRT patch and told that my own GP had done me a great disservice by not helping me. Unfortunately I struggled with the patches as they did not adhere well to my skin, but I then went back to my own practice and saw a different GP, who immediately put me on HRT tablets. Within about ten days I could feel the difference and I have not had anxiety since. I have also not had any hot flushes and generally feel much happier in myself. The only side effect from the tablets has been a bit of weight gain and a sensation of heavy breasts – both of which I can live with.' **Dina, 53**

Dina is correct: the 2015 NICE guidelines *do* advocate HRT as a treatment option for psychological symptoms. Specifically, the recommendation is that doctors consider HRT to alleviate low mood that arises as a result of menopause along with CBT[2], which we'll come onto in Chapter 6.

'Wahey! I'm off to the doctor to get a prescription!' you might respond, and with such marked benefits, who could blame you? But hold your horses a moment, because HRT is only one option and we're here to guide you through other treatments available to you. So before you opt for HRT, it's worth being aware of the bigger picture.

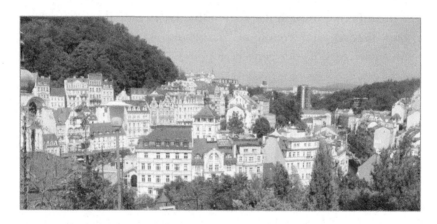

5.3 What are the drawbacks?

So, let's go back in time to the 1990s, when the odds are you were not even *thinking* about your periods stopping. (I don't know about you, but I was far too preoccupied with dancing on nightclub podiums, dating unsuitable men and slaving away in an ad agency to pay much attention to where I'd be at twenty years hence. Oops, I digress.) For many decades, until 2002, HRT was very widely prescribed across the western world. Then, in close succession, came the publication of two reports which cast doubt on its usage.

The first was the **Women's Health Initiative** in 2002. Compared to any studies that had gone before, the WHI was huge. It involved 16,000 postmenopausal women, and looked at the impact of HRT over a period of eight and a half years. The main issue was that the study failed to verify that HRT helped reduce the risk of heart attacks and strokes as had previously been believed. Also, it suggested there was a link between HRT and an increased risk of breast cancer.

Then, in 2003, came the **Million Women Study.** This national study of women's health **was** a collaborative project between Cancer Research UK and the National Health Service, and involved more than one million UK women aged 50 and over. This appeared to confirm the relationship between HRT and the risk of breast cancer, and implicated HRT in endometrial and ovarian cancer too.

In the wake of this research, to say there was concern about HRT is an understatement. Prescriptions halved almost overnight. Overall the number of women taking HRT fell by 66%. Since the early noughties, elements of both studies have been called into question. Yet this retraction of some of the previous findings received little publicity in the media. For example as recently as 2015, when a report came out relating to ovarian cancer, the BBC, which tends to be more circumspect, had a headline: 'HRT increases ovarian cancer risk'. Whilst it's true that the University of Oxford research published in *The Lancet* showed a rise in ovarian cancer risk for women taking HRT, what it revealed is not as alarming as the BBC headline. Taking HRT for five years is linked to one extra case of ovarian cancer per 1,000 women, which takes expected incidence from 20 women in 1,000 to 21 per 1,000. According to Professor Montserrat Garcia-Closas from the Institute of Cancer Research in London, the latest data shows a modest increase in a relatively uncommon cancer, and she feels that for a woman of average risk, then breast cancer will remain a more important consideration than ovarian cancer.

5.4 Weighing up the pros and cons

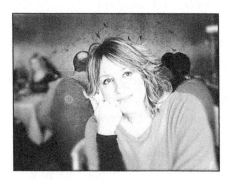

The job of this guide is just that – to *guide* you – and so rather than swamp you with information as to what's been proven and disproven, here, very broadly, is the current position on HRT and breast cancer:

- According to Cancer Research UK, any personal or family history of breast cancer rules out the possibility of using HRT, unless it's absolutely clear that the cancer was non-hormonally linked. On rare occasions GPs will refer you to a gynaecologist if your family history is complex and you have very bad menopausal symptoms.
- Cancer Research UK also states there may be a small increased risk of breast cancer cells being stimulated and hence breast cancer being diagnosed *if certain types of HRT are used for more than five years after the age of 50.*
- It's important to note **that there is no evidence of an increased risk of breast cancer in women on HRT under the age of 50 compared with menstruating women of the same age.**
- The age of the woman at the time of starting treatment therefore makes a difference to the risk factors.
- The good news for women already taking HRT is that risks seem to return to normal five years after stopping.
- However, it should be noted that regardless of the type of HRT, by any standards, a 0.08% increased risk of breast cancer for each year of HRT use (which is what was revealed in the WHI) is extremely low.

- Some think that the type of progestogen used may make a difference. Research is ongoing, and aims to find the most 'breast-friendly' hormones.
- Drinking two or more units of alcohol per day or being overweight are greater risks for diagnosis of breast cancer than taking HRT for five years after the age of 50.

In other words, the risks of developing breast cancer as a result of HRT are relative, and depend on a number of factors. It's also worth noting that whilst the risks of breast, ovarian and endometrial cancers become marginally higher, it appears the risk of heart disease may go down. (For a summary of the latest findings visit **www.evidentlycochrane.net**.) It's worth considering that **the route of delivery of oestrogen is also believed to have an impact.** Oestrogen delivered through skin patches or gel has a lower risk of causing stroke or blood clots than oral HRT because it breaks down more slowly.

In addition, research compiled over the last ten years means **HRT is now considered effective for the prevention of postmenopausal osteoporosis,** but only whilst you are taking it. Bone density will decrease rapidly after HRT is stopped, so, HRT is generally recommended only for women at significant risk, for whom non-oestrogen therapies are unsuitable.

Whilst hormone replacement therapy may be useful, the risks and benefits of treatment must be considered for each individual, say NICE. They list drawbacks as:

- Oestrogen-related adverse effects – fluid retention, bloating, breast tenderness, nausea, headaches, leg cramps and dyspepsia
- Progestogen-related adverse effects – mood swings, depression, fluid retention, breast tenderness, headaches or migraine, acne and lower abdominal pain. These resemble the side effects some experience when taking the pill, so may be familiar to you anyway!
- Bleeding

The NICE position is that:

- HRT has not been shown to increase cardiovascular disease when started in women aged under 60 years of age, or affect the risk of dying from cardiovascular disease.
- HRT is not associated with an increased risk of developing type 2 diabetes.
- Oestrogen-only HRT has little or no increase in the risk of breast cancer. HRT with oestrogen and progestogen can be associated with an increase in the risk of breast cancer but any increase risk reduces after stopping HRT.

You can read the Royal College of Obstetricians and Gynaecologists and British Menopause Association's review of the 2002 WHI clinical trial at www.rcog.org.uk/en/news/rcogbms-response-to-review-of-hrt-study/ and there is further exploration of the risks and benefits of HRT on **www.patient.co.uk**.

I think you'll agree what's emerging is that HRT is a case of 'swings and roundabouts'. Each woman has to weigh up the advantages and disadvantages of the treatment for herself, and follow the path that feels right for her.

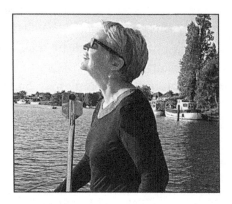

5.5 Different types of HRT

As the name implies, hormone replacement therapy replaces the hormones that a woman's body is no longer producing due to the menopause, i.e.

- **Oestrogen** – which is taken either from plants or the urine of pregnant horses (more on this shortly). The oestrogen used in HRT is not as strong as the oestrogen in the contraceptive pill.
- **Progesterone** – HRT uses a synthetic version of progesterone called progestogen, which is easier for the body to absorb.

The fact that 50 different preparations of HRT are now available should make it easier to find a fitting solution for each woman, but the choice can seem overwhelming. It may find it helpful if we divide HRT into the following types. You can see similar breakdown on www.nhs.co.uk.

1. If you start HRT **when you are still having periods,** or have just finished periods you will normally be advised to use a cyclical combined HRT preparation. There are two types:
   - **Monthly cyclical HRT,** which is normally advised for women who have menopausal symptoms but who are still having regular periods. With this, you take oestrogen every day, but progestogen is added in for 14 days of each 28-day treatment cycle. This causes a regular bleed (loss of the lining of the womb, but not a period as such, because HRT does not cause ovulation) every 28 days.
   - **Three-monthly cyclical HRT** is sometimes advised for women who have menopausal symptoms but are having very irregular periods. Here you take oestrogen every day, then you also take progestogen for 14 days, every 13 weeks. This means that you have a bleed every three months. However this uses less progestogen than the monthly option so offers less protection against endometrial cancer. The **Mirena coil** is also an option if you have bleed issues.

2. **If you've had no period for a year or more, you're considered to be postmenopausal,** so if you start HRT at this point, you will normally be advised to take a continuous combined HRT preparation. This means that you will take both oestrogen and progestogen every day. The dose and type of these hormones is finely balanced so don't usually cause a monthly bleed.

In both instances, you and your doctor might like to discuss using the IUS (intrauterine system) or Mirena coil (which is also licensed for heavy periods) as the progestogen part of HRT. You will need to add oestrogen as a tablet, gel or patch, but according to NICE guidelines, transdermal (patches) and IUS HRT have lower risk factors than oral HRT. Further details can be found at **www.nice.org.uk/news/ article/women-with-symptoms-of-menopause-should-not-suffer-in-silence.**

3. **If you have had a hysterectomy,** you will only need to take HRT that contains oestrogen. The progestogen is added in to other types of HRT so that the lining of the uterus does not build up, so, if your uterus has been totally removed, progestogen is not needed.

4. **If you mainly have genital symptoms** such as vaginal dryness (which we will talk more of in Chapter 8) you may choose to try some vaginal oestrogen cream or pessaries. These are often sufficient to relieve symptoms.

Please note that **it is *not* a good idea to be on any form of the treatment indefinitely,** (which is unfortunate if it's worked for you). **NICE also recommend that any HRT treatment should be reviewed at three months, and that women should aim to take the lowest dose, for the least amount of time.**

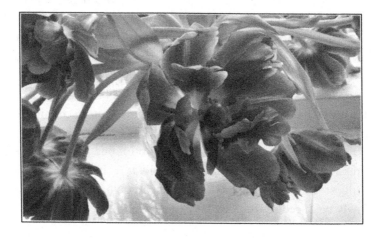

Sarah: What are Bio-Identical Hormones? Women like Oprah Winfrey and Jeanette Winterson seem to have had very positive experiences with them.

Patrick: Well, this certainly *is* a hot topic! The phrase 'Bio-Identical Hormone Therapy' first began to be used widely as a marketing term for custom-mixed hormones which became popular in the wake of the Women's Health Initiative in 2002. Many of my colleagues in the medical profession are cynical about the value of custom-mixed hormones, because the suppliers who mix these compounds often rely on salivary and blood tests to 'assess' hormone levels, yet as we've already discussed, these tests are pretty meaningless for midlife women. Hormone levels vary from day to day, even hour to hour. Moreover, although the idea of a custom-mixed hormone sounds appealing, research has shown the practice can have an adverse effect.

These days the term 'Bio-Identical Hormones' is more usually used to refer to compounds that are plant based and have the same chemical and molecular structure as hormones that are produced in the female body, and with this comes an implication that these hormones are natural and more benign. Strictly speaking, *all* hormones are synthesised in a laboratory from some precursor by the action of enzymes. It's also claimed that bio-identical hormones are different from conventional hormone regimens and will prevent disease, which as yet remains unproven.

Bio-Identical Hormones are not available through your NHS GP, but if you care about animal welfare, it is worth noting that certain drugs used in synthetic HRT – Prempak-C, Prempro, Premique, Premarin or the combined menopausal-osteoporosis drug Duavee (formerly known as Aprela) – contain conjugated horse oestrogen. They are synthesized from urine, and, according to Peta, in order to extract the urine, mares are kept in small stalls unable to move much or lie down. If you'd prefer to avoid non-equine products, you can ask your GP to prescribe a different product; Femoston /Prognova or Nuvelle (which are soya based) or Climaval (which is synthetic), for example. If he or she is reluctant to accommodate you ask for a referral to a Menopause Clinic or a Gynae-Endocrine Consultant at a hospital.

As a male doctor, I'd be the first to acknowledge that you know what it feels like to go through the menopause and I don't, so the ultimate decision has to rest with the patient. If you do decide to pursue this route, however, just keep in mind that long-term studies regarding safety of bio-identical hormones are scarce. Until proven otherwise, the risks of getting a cancer with Bio-Identical Hormones remain the same as synthetic HRT, and neither form of treatment should be used over an extended period of time.

In the meantime, I suggest reading about Jeanette's experience in *The Guardian* and the US Food and Drug Adminstration's advice to consumers for insight into opposing views. The links are at the end of this book.

5.7 The final decision is yours

In weighing up the options, don't forget that *all* medication is associated with some risk, even aspirin, and in many circumstances taking *no* medication has enormous drawbacks. (Let's not forget what advances in medicine have given us, please. I don't wish to return to the days before anesthetics, for instance, and my hunch is you won't either.) We may never have a perfect type of hormone replacement, but with better understanding of the benefits and actual risks, it is hoped that more women can access accurate information to help them make informed choices about whether or not to use HRT.

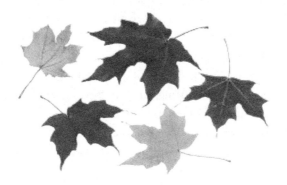

'As someone who has always been pill averse, I never thought I would take HRT. However, after months of hot flushes, sleeplessness and generally feeling dreadful, I decided I could suffer in silence no longer (though my husband may not agree with the silence bit). The first two HRT formulations I tried didn't work for me. While they made me feel better, they also made me bleed heavily (which negates one of the only advantages of the menopause). Finally, after much to-ing and fro-ing to the doctors, I have found one that suits. For me the plus sides of HRT definitely outweigh the risks, although I understand why others feel differently. Each woman must do what's best for her and her lifestyle.' **Trish, 58**

'I've always been a bit of an insomniac, but when the menopause hit me, and I do mean **hit**, I couldn't bear the hideous night sweats at all. HRT helped with that, so when my doctor refused to extend it, I was devastated. I'd been on it for nearly 10 years, and was then prescribed patches of HRT which caused more problems than the cure. I'm now not on anything (having tried natural remedies, which were ineffective) and have all the original symptoms of menopause: hot flushes, insomnia, emotional lows and general malaise. I'm tempted to buy my original HRT from the internet, but know it could be dodgy. I'm going back to my doctor but hold little hope for help or a referral. The general attitude seems to be "get on with it".' **Stella, 58**

If you *do* opt for HRT, your treatment plan should be tailored to you. **Before going to see your doctor, I suggest you review your own situation and it might be a good idea to write some notes.** You may like to consider:

- **Why are you taking HRT?**
  - Is it for perimenopausal/menopausal symptoms?
  - Is it to protect against heart disease and/or osteoporosis?
- If you are considering HRT to relieve physical symptoms such as hot flushes or night sweats, **take the severity of your symptoms into account.**
  - How much discomfort and distress are they causing you?
  - Are they interfering with your daily life in a major way? (See 'Seeking Medical Advice' in Chapter 1 as a guide.)
- **The same is true of psychological symptoms.**

- If you're anxious, does your anxiety prevent you from carrying out your usual day-to-day activities?
- Is your depression affecting your relationships and ability to work?
- **Where are you are in terms of the menopause?**
  - Have you stopped menstruating?
  - If so, when?
- **Your age is a factor too.**
  - Have you experienced an early or premature menopause?

Once you've got to grips with this, you'll be well equipped to chat your circumstances through with your doctor. Together you are far better placed to work out what's right for you than Patrick or I will ever be. Your GP will also consider:

- Your medical history
- Other medication you are on
- Your family history: is there a history of breast cancer in your family?

In making your decision, it's possible that you might find it helpful to track your situation in the 'Decision Making Tree' on **www.menopausematters.co.uk** although be prepared for it to take a while because the subject is complicated.

Overall, it could be said that the biggest argument in HRT's favour is that if you're a woman with severe symptoms, it often *works*. There are alternatives (see Chapter 6) but, as Ken Muse, MD, from the University of Kentucky writes in Medscape, although problems have been shown to improve when patients use some non-hormonal prescription drugs and herbs, women with significant symptoms are seldom as satisfied with these as with HRT.

5.7 Coming off HRT

'I went cold turkey and stopped HRT. A year on, I was suffering hot flushes, which was bad, but bearable. What I didn't expect was the panic attack I

experienced on, of all things, a massage table. That did it. I went straight to my doctor and resumed my prescription. No more panic attacks, and – wonderfully – no more hot flushes, immediately. If I got my way, I'd <u>never</u> come off HRT!' **Susie, 57**

When you decide to come off HRT, it should be done gradually. I made the mistake of suddenly stopping antidepressants many years ago, and it was *awful*. I completely lost my marbles for a few days and didn't know which way was up. Whilst antidepressants and HRT are not the same, they are similar in that both impact our hormones and going cold turkey with either is a bad idea. If you come off HRT overnight, this can be very stressful for your body, which will have become used to the additional supply of oestrogen.

<u>Q&A</u>

Sarah: Does HRT simply delay the onset of menopausal symptoms until you stop taking it?

Patrick: If you come off HRT gradually having been on it for a few years, you may have a relapse of menopausal symptoms although these should pass within a few months. To avoid this happening, I tend to advise patients to reduce the dose over 3-6 months. I'd then suggest staying off the treatment completely for 2-3 months to give your hormones a chance to settle. If symptoms remain severe several months after stopping, then restarting treatment is probably the best course of action. Although there are no guarantees, hopefully a lower dose than was initially prescribed will prove effective at this point, and you can then cease HRT at a later date.

According to Dame Dr Shirley Bond, if HRT is stopped suddenly the oestrogen levels will drop quickly to low levels. She advises that you wean yourself off, gradually reducing the dosage. The ways in which you do this will depend on the sort of HRT you are taking, so you should also consult your doctor to work out the best way forward.

The truth is that since there is no way of foreseeing how long oestrogen withdrawal symptoms last, **there is no way of predicting**

how long you will need HRT to continue to control symptoms. In this respect HRT is not an exact science. Some women may choose to take it for a year or two, others for longer; the management plan is down to the individual. But if you do decide to take HRT, **ongoing yearly reviews with your doctor are essential.** Then you can discuss the appropriate type, dose and route that will maximize benefits and minimize risk for as long as you continue to take it.

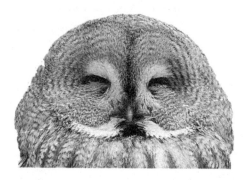

'Let men be wise by instinct if they can, but when this fails, be wise by good advice.' **Sophocles**

6.   'A' is for Alternatives to HRT

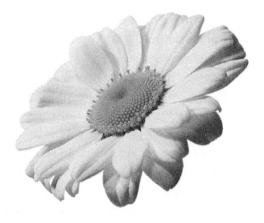

There's not space in this book to examine *all* the alternative ways to treat menopausal symptoms aside from HRT, so what follows is a broad overview of the options, some of which you may wish to explore further.

HRT is not for every woman, and for a number of reasons. For many of us, the benefits of using HRT don't outweigh the drawbacks: perhaps our symptoms aren't severe enough for us to feel the risks, however low, are worth it; or perhaps HRT is off the agenda for health reasons. We've already mentioned that a personal or family history of breast, endometrial or ovarian cancer almost always precludes the use of HRT, and HRT is not recommended for women with a history of liver disease or a heart condition, either. If you have high blood pressure, that would have to be brought under control first.

Yet unfortunately a history of other diseases like these doesn't preclude you from menopausal symptoms – 65-85% of breast cancer patients will suffer from hot flushes and night sweats, for instance. As a result, **many women are keen to find safe, effective non-hormonal treatments**. Should you decide to pursue a non-pharmaceutical route, you would be far from alone: around 30% of women consider alternatives to HRT to combat their symptoms. Others simply feel that an 'alternative' approach sits more comfortably with them for ethical, cultural or personal reasons. But first, let's have a quick look at medication your GP might offer you instead of HRT.

6.1 Pharmaceutical alternatives to HRT

- **Tibolone is a synthetic hormone that mimics the activity of oestrogen and progesterone.** It is only suitable for women who have been through the menopause and whose uterus is intact, but in these circumstances it can help to restore the balance of female hormones and thus ease the distress caused by continuing hot flushes and night sweats. Tibolone is also prescribed to help prevent osteoporosis (bone loss – a subject we'll return to in Chapter 7). If, however, you are unable to take HRT for medical reasons, you will probably not be able to take tibolone either.

- **There are several antidepressant medications which may be effective in treating hot flushes,** including venlafaxine and citalopram, but the main reason you may choose to explore antidepressants as an option is that **they can help lessen anxiety and depression.** If you feel that hormone fluctuations and/or your circumstances are having such a negative impact on your mood that you can no longer function day to day, it's worth talking to your GP. Be forewarned, however; most antidepressants take several weeks to work so you will have to be patient before you experience any benefits, and initially you may suffer side effects.

- **Clonidine** is a medicine originally designed to treat high blood pressure which used to be thought helpful in reducing hot flushes and night sweats. Whilst it may still benefit those taking it, there are more effective medications available with fewer side effects.

- **Gabapentin** is chiefly used to treat nerve pain, but **in the short term has been shown to decrease the frequency of hot flushes by 45-71%.** Adverse effects can be common during the first 1-2 weeks of treatment and include drowsiness, unsteadiness and dizziness.

Your doctor will be able to advise you more fully on all these, and there's further information on **www.patient.co.uk**.

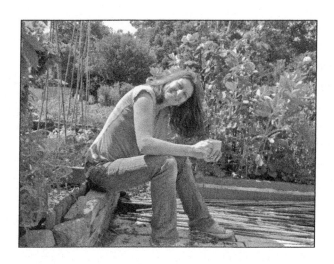

6.2 The pros and cons of alternative treatment

If you wish to manage the menopause without the aid of pharmaceutical medicine that has to be prescribed by your GP, there are many doors open to you. We've already touched on dozens of ways you can help yourself feel better in terms of practical tips, managing your diet and exercise. But in addition to this, there are many complementary medicines and treatments on offer for menopause-related symptoms.

'I'd had poor experiences with western medicine in the past, and knew I didn't want to take chemicals, so from the off I decided to pursue an alternative route. During the early stages of perimenopause I had regular massages and now I see an acupuncturist in the way others might see a regular doctor. I've used him as my baseline for advice and to discuss where I am at and how well I feel and he's been trying to redress the balance of my hormones. I also see a herbalist who specialises in this field. Together we look at supporting my cycle and the elements my body is missing with Chinese herbs.' **Holly, 54**

What should you choose?

Alternative approaches you might like to consider include:
- Acupuncture

- Chiropractic
- Cognitive Behavioural Therapy
- Herbal remedies
- Homeopathy
- Massage therapy
- Mindfulness Meditation
- Reiki
- Traditional Chinese Medicine

We'll look at several of these presently.

*'As for what kind of therapy to go for? I'd say **listen to yourself**. In our society we're told doctors know everything and we know nothing, but actually **you** are the best expert on your body that you know. If you're attracted to a certain kind of therapy, explore it. Read up about it first, and then, if it resonates, seek a recommendation from someone whose opinion you respect. There's a lot of mystery attached to some of these practices, but often they aren't that mysterious.'* **Holly, 54**

If you discover an avenue that piques your interest, like Holly, I'm all for exploring it. I don't feel it's my place to discourage anyone from finding alternative ways of gaining support. All I offer is a few guidelines and insights – the rest is down to you as an individual. You might like to have a look at the Decision Making Tree on www.menopausematters.co.uk to help you plan a way forward.

Working with your body

One of the most appealing aspects of alternative approaches such as acupuncture, Traditional Chinese Medicine, massage therapy and chiropractic is that **therapists aim to work *with* your body**. Perhaps it's because many of these disciplines have different cultural origins to western medicine. Acupuncturist and herbalist Cathy Margolin says that traditionally Asian cultures don't turn to artificial hormone remedies by default in the way we tend to in Britain and America. Instead they appear to have an inherent understanding that food and herbs can be added to the daily diet to help manage these changes when they first occur.

*'With both my acupuncturist and my herbalist, in my initial appointment, we discussed who I was, what I did and what I am normally like when well. Above all, I didn't get medicalized. I didn't get told I was **ill**. I like that approach – to be treated as a whole person. We can have discussions of "I'm in this place in my life..." so I don't feel I'm being told something is wrong, there's no negativity. It's not about "take this pill and the symptoms will go away." It's about supporting me through this difficult, challenging experience.'* **Holly, 54**

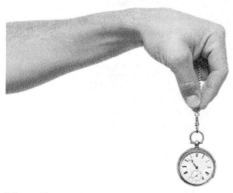

More time

There can be another positive aspect to alternative therapy: **one of the things you tend to get – and this is no small thing – is time.** There's very little alternative therapy that is available for menopausal symptoms on the NHS (there is a remote possibility of CBT, but it tends to be postcode lottery, and your GP is more likely to refer you to a consultant gynaecologist). At least paying for a private consultation means you tend to get more than ten minutes, which is what a GP is allocated for each patient.

'With a reputable alternative practitioner, I find you invariably have an hour as your first appointment. They listen to your story and get the whole picture of your body changes – your symptoms, your emotions, your work, your creativity – all of it.' **Juliet, 53**

Finding a reputable practitioner

So far, so enticing. The problem with alternative therapies is how to sort the wheat from the chaff, or more precisely, the charlatans from the conscientious practitioners. Conventional medicine is controlled by statutory regulation to help ensure that doctors are properly qualified and adhere to certain codes of practice.

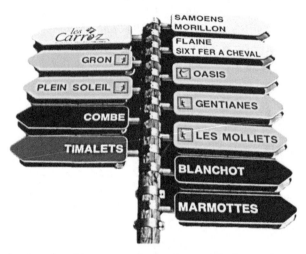

Professionals of two complementary and alternative treatments – osteopathy and chiropractic – are regulated in a similar way. But there is no statutory professional regulation of any other complementary and alternative medicine (CAM) here in the UK, which can leave patients open to the possibility of malpractice.

Your safest bet is to check that your therapist is registered with an organisation that is itself registered with the Professional Standards Authority – as is the case for anyone listed with the Complementary and Natural Healthcare Council or the British Acupuncture Council. Other professional associations hold membership lists or registers of practitioners of specific complementary and alternative medicines, such as the British Homeopathic Association, The Reiki Association and the UK Register of Chinese Herbal Medicine.

As to whether alternative therapy *works*, I fear that to enter into this argument is to open a can of proverbial worms. I could give you my opinion, (and so could Patrick), but it would be subjective. Instead

I've included links to trials and research where I could find them which back up the efficacy of the treatments listed. If you're interested in reading more about what western science has established about alternative therapies, this link is a good place to start. However, you may be sceptical about western science and its methodology and prefer to trust your intuition. On the whole I'd say that, if a treatment is working for you and you can afford it, continue, because your wellbeing is the most important thing of all.

6.3 Herbal Remedies

A number of herbs have been explored as potential treatments for menopausal symptoms. Among the most popular, the most promising in terms of effectiveness seem to be:

- **Black cohosh**: Studies in Europe found black cohosh may provide symptomatic relief of menopausal hot flushes, night sweats, insomnia, nervousness and irritability because it has an oestrogen-like activity within the body although large-scale research has yet to be done. There are a number of Black Cohosh products on the market for menopause including Remifemin, which is marketed as 'the safe, natural alternative to HRT'. It has been associated with liver toxicity, however, so is best not taken over the long term.
- **Ginseng:** This is a herb which has been used for its therapeutic health benefits for thousands of years by the Chinese, Koreans, and Native Americans. It may help to treat menopausal symptoms of fatigue, anxiety and stress because it's considered a 'normalizer and an energizer' and a trial using red ginseng has demonstrated efficacy. You can take ginseng in different forms including tea, powder, and extract.
- **Red clover**: According to research published by the Journal of the British Menopause Society, red clover supplements, used in controlled studies, may have a positive effect on the rate of bone loss, improve cardiovascular health, and offer some protective effect against breast and endometrial cancer. This is because it

contains phytoestrogens – plant substances that have a similar effect to oestrogen, of which the most important groups are isoflavones and lignans. According to the BMS, 'The role of phytoestrogens has stimulated considerable interest since populations consuming a diet high in isoflavones such as the Japanese appear to have lower rates of menopausal vasomotor symptoms, heart disease, osteoporosis; breast, colon, endometrial and ovarian cancers.'

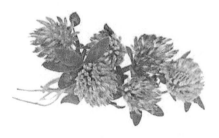

- **Pine bark:** One small Japanese study found that pine bark supplement helped relieve hot flushes as well as other menopause-related symptoms.
- **St. John's Wort:** Among the most popular herbs in the UK and US, St. John's Wort has long been an alternative treatment for menopausal mood swings, improved sleep, relaxation, and reduced depression and anxiety. Derived from a wild flowering plant called *Hypericum perforatum*, the leaves and flowers are harvested and dried. They can then be brewed in a tea or taken in a pill or liquid form. Scientific studies affirm that while St. John's Wort is effective for treating mild depression, it works no better than a placebo for treating severe depression.
- **Folic acid:** Of all supplements, this seems to be one of the most effective at improving hot flushes according to a number of trials. One study from University of Alexandria showed a 65% reduction if the dosage was maintained over a number of weeks, and once women stopped taking folic acid, the hot flushes returned.

You also might like to look into **Sage leaf extract** and **Evening Primrose Oil**.

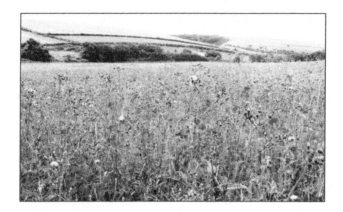

A word of caution

Many women choose to try herbal products as they believe them to be safer than prescribed medication. They are often labeled as 'natural', which sounds appealing but reveals little in terms of how these products are actually made; NICE guidelines state that clinicians should 'Explain to women who wish to try complementary therapies that the quality, purity and constituents of products may be unknown'. It's important to be aware that many herbal products available in the UK are not subject to the same degree of standardization, which means there may be variability between products or a lack of clarity regarding ingredients. This can also make it difficult to compare trial results.

What to look for

The best way through this confusion is to:

- Look out for **Traditional Herbal Registration (THR) marking on the product packaging**. This means the herbal remedy has been assessed against quality standards, and you'll have information about how and when to use it. THR products do not require the supervision of a medical practitioner and you can find them in your local health shop, pharmacy or supermarket (there will be a THR number on the packet).

- **Avoid buying herbal medications online** because herbal medicines manufactured outside the UK may not be subject to regulation.
- Be aware that **some herbal medicines and pharmaceutical products don't work well in conjunction**. Some types of antidepressants shouldn't be combined with St. John's Wort, for instance, so please check with your GP before you combine any of them.

6.4 Traditional Chinese Medicine

'I went to my (female) doctor when I was 42. I had not had regular periods for a while, was exhausted, depressed, anxious and had awful itching all over my body. She told me I was too young to even be going through the perimenopause. I went from pillar to post – dermatologists, counselling, and had lots of time off work. Finally, in despair, I went to my local Chinese Medical Centre where instantly I was told I was in perimenopause, given acupuncture and told how to manage my condition as best I could.' **Kerry, 45**

In China, the ancient herbal system of medicine still forms a major part of healthcare provision and is made available in state hospitals alongside western medicine. The tradition goes right back to the 3rd century BC, and in its broadest sense Chinese medicine includes herbal therapy, acupuncture, dietary therapy and exercises in breathing and movement (tai chi and qi gong). Some or several of these may be employed in the course of treatment.

Chinese Herbal Medicine, along with the other components of Chinese medicine, is based on the concepts of yin and yang. It aims to understand and treat the many ways in which the fundamental balance and harmony between the two may be undermined and the ways in which a person's Qi or vitality may be depleted or blocked. Specific symptoms are believed to reflect an imbalance of Qi, and clinical strategies are based upon diagnosis of these indicators.

Practitioners of Traditional Chinese Medicine argue that this ancient methodology can help **prevent or reduce the severity of nearly all of your menopausal symptoms** rather than just relieving them temporarily. According to acupuncturist and herbalist Cathy Margolin, menopausal symptoms are essentially a deficiency in kidney yin and yang: yang is the energy of movement and represents daytime and heat, she says, whereas yin is the energy of stillness, nighttime and coolness. Stress and ageing damage our yin, which can result in night sweats and insomnia as menopause approaches, but menopause can also exhibit itself as a deficiency of kidney yang energy. In this case both energies need balancing and nourishing.

For more on Traditional Chinese Medicine and a list of qualified practitioners see **www.rchm.co.uk**.

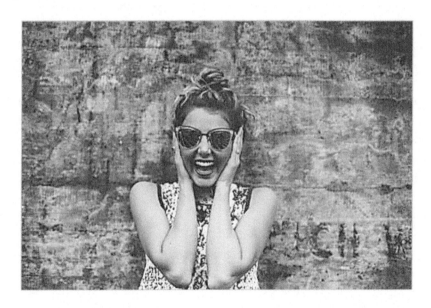

'I'm not going to accept a hard, masculine, medicalized style of approach. I prefer a gentler, holistic style of treatment that takes time, that's about rhythms and the cycles of life After all, that's what we're going through – the menopause is the most natural thing in the world. It's important to honour that and look after ourselves. We don't have to be out there striving to sort it instantly. During this change we have to honour the transformation. And what's why I want to go through this naturally.' **Holly, 54**

6.5 Acupuncture

Many women have gained relief from their menopause symptoms through acupuncture. It involves the usually painless process of placing extremely thin needles into the skin along specific 'acupuncture points'. **Acupuncturists view these points as nodes where lines of bodily energy converge. The needles help to open any blockages and balance your body gently back to health.** Usually a series of treatments is needed to get the best results, and the amount suggested is revealed after the first exam and treatment.

Although these lines of energy do not correspond to any actual physical structures known to western medicine and skeptics argue that acupuncture benefits are the result of the placebo effect, research has now confirmed that acupuncture is a reasonable alternative to hormone therapy for women suffering from menopausal depression and hot flushes. A recent study found that women who received traditional Chinese acupuncture had less severe hot flushes and mood swings than women receiving a placebo treatment, and past research found that acupuncture worked as well as the antidepressant venlafaxine (Effexor), when treating hot flushes in women after breast cancer treatment. Not only did the acupuncture cause no negative side effects (while venlafaxine caused nausea, fatigue, anxiety and more), but its effects, which also included increased energy, sex drive and a sense of wellbeing, lasted for 15 weeks longer.

'Acupuncture is the weirdest sensation. When my acupuncturist hits the right point, it's not remotely like being jabbed by a sewing needle or having an injection. Instead it's like a jolt of electricity – a whoosh! – and I can feel the release of energy. Once, when I was having very bad anxiety, I spent the whole session with needles in my feet, which surprisingly didn't hurt. The practitioner said that she was bringing my energy out of my upper body and back down to take me out of my head and reground me. When I tried to run the next day, my feet felt like bricks, they were so heavy, but the sensation of panic had lifted. I've no idea how or why it works, but it seems to.' **Juliet, 53**

6.6 Cognitive Behavioural Therapy

Although Cognitive Behavioural Therapy (CBT) tends to be thought of as a psychological therapy (I mentioned it in Chapter 2, in relation to anxiety) it's often used to help with physical health problems. One of the benefits is that **it promotes the understanding that thoughts, emotions, behaviours and physical responses are linked, and thus connects the mind and body.** In this respect it mirrors traditional holistic treatments like acupuncture.

We've already seen that we don't exactly know how hot flushes work, but we do know stress seems to make them worse. Professor Myra Hunter of the Institute of Psychiatry at Kings College London would doubtless agree: her research, recently published in *The Lancet*, showed that CBT can reduce the impact of hot flushes and night sweats. Women given weekly CBT reported that their discomfort had significantly diminished nine weeks after starting therapy; they were more able to cope with their symptoms too. At six months they still found the hot flushes and night sweats less of a problem, and their mood, sleep patterns and quality of life had all improved.

Professor Hunter says that, as **with any physical symptoms, the way we manage them can make a difference**. You probably recall that in Chapter 3 we mentioned that deep breathing exercises can help to lessen the impact of a flush and women who wake up due to night sweats are more likely to go back to sleep if they learn how to remain calm rather than getting distressed. The breath gives us something to focus on, and helps to counter negative thoughts.

If CBT appeals to you, the British Association of Behavioural and Cognitive Psychotherapies (**www.babcp.com**) lists accredited counsellors.

6.7 Mindfulness meditation

One of the biggest buzzwords in psychotherapeutic circles is 'mindfulness'. Put simply, mindfulness entails focusing your mind on the present moment rather than the past or the future, and in this respect reflects much more ancient Buddhist teachings.

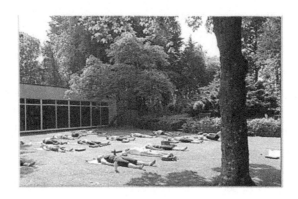

Its proponents say that we can spend so much of our time going over the past or worrying about the future that we end up missing much of the richness of the life we have right now. Mindfulness practice offers the opportunity to wake up to our lives in this moment, which can help us to live with greater presence, aliveness, clarity and enjoyment.

Mindfulness meditation, which can be used in conjunction with CBT, has been shown to reduce stress and anxiety and NICE now recommends mindfulness-based courses for people with recurrent depression. **Mindfulness can also be used to alleviate the distress of pain, and thus help manage physical menopausal symptoms, and research also shows that mindfulness practices can help with insomnia in postmenopausal women.**

For more information, see **www.bemindful.co.uk.**

'Shortly after I had a partial hysterectomy, I went into the full-on menopause. Although I'd had mild perimenopausal symptoms before, I had hot flushes like I'd never experienced before – sweat would pour off me at the most inopportune moments and I had to carry a fan and towel at all times. The night sweats got worse, and I still sleep with a towel over my pillow so I can mop my face in the night. I've always been plump, but I put on weight, particularly round my middle. I wondered why I was so exhausted all the time, and aged 50 I suffered an episode of severe depression and anxiety.

It was then that I discovered mindfulness. I am now 52 and still have many of the same symptoms of the menopause but am much better able to deal with them. I am on antidepressants which help, I had a course of Cognitive

Behavioural Therapy, I cycle regularly and practice yoga and meditation. Whilst I still get tired if I overdo it, I am now much better at managing my energy levels, managing my health (physical and mental) and not letting symptoms overwhelm me.' **Vicky, 52**

6.8 Yoga and pilates

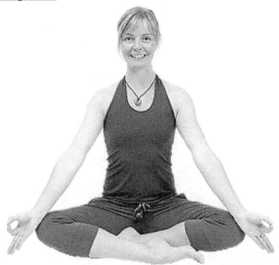

© yogaforyou.uk.com

When our hormones are fluctuating wildly, it can leave us feeling out of balance physically and emotionally. On a rough day, I've felt victim to my changing body, tired, achy and old before my time. **Yoga exercises can help level out this sense of physiological instability by relaxing and gently stretching every muscle**, promoting better blood circulation and oxygen supply to cells and tissues. Yoga can also improve the health of the digestive tract, nervous system and other organs. And at a time when we're often prone to exhaustion and feel muggy-headed and clumsy, it can increase energy and improve balance, thus giving us back a sense of power and control. But don't just take my word for it – there's evidence to support the notion that yoga can help relieve menopausal symptoms such as hot flushes and sleep disturbance, as well as irritability and depression. If yoga appeals to you and you've not tried it before, start with a class once or twice a week. Once you learn the basics, perhaps you can carve out some personal time to practise in the comfort of your own home.

Alternatively, **you might like to try Pilates, which offers many of the benefits of yoga as it also focuses on developing strength, balance, flexibility, posture and good breathing technique**. However it tends to have much less emphasis on spiritual practices and meditation, which may – or may not – appeal to you.

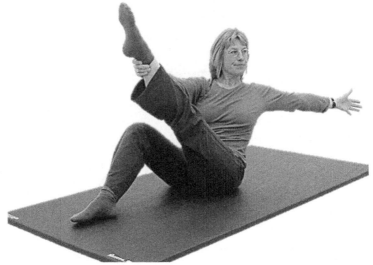

©airevalleypilates.co.uk

6.9 Alexander Technique

If **you'd like to improve fluidity of movement and overall wellbeing, you might like to look into Alexander technique.**

'I was perimenopausal when I began my training to become an Alexander technique teacher, and I honestly don't know how I would have coped otherwise (my GP wouldn't put me on HRT, apparently because of my weight). So many of the symptoms (anxiety, mood swings, anger and irritability, body image, muscular aches and pains, hot flushes, sleep problems etc.) can be helped by learning what Alexander technique teachers teach.

Many people think that it's 'about posture' when it is so much more than this, although good posture is one of the benefits; to summarize, what I learned over my 3-year course is to teach people how to be less tense, less

120

reactive and more 'present'. Obviously Alexander technique can help anyone at any age and in any walk of life, but in my own experience this can only have positive effects on all of those menopause symptoms. I recommend it to anyone who is willing to consider changing their habits to improve their function and ease (mental and physical). It's available around the country and is a worthwhile and enjoyable investment, if not a quick fix.' **Pia, 53**

A major benefit that yoga, Pilates and Alexander Technique share is that they all focus on strengthening the pelvic floor. Whether you've given birth or not, the decrease in oestrogen which comes with the menopause may initiate thinning and weakening of the pelvic muscles. This makes us more susceptible to decreased tone, elasticity and suppleness in the tissues of the pelvic floor. Strengthening your pelvic floor prior to and during this time of transition is a win-win: helping to ensure comfort and pleasurable sex throughout the years, and minimizing the chances of urinary and/or stool incontinence later in life.

6.10 Massage

People have used massage to promote relaxation, improve blood flow, ease tension and relieve pain for thousands of years. Archeological evidence has been found in many ancient civilizations all over the world – and it remains popular today.

There are many types of massage. Some are gentle, some intense. With a Swedish massage the therapist will use long, gliding strokes along with kneading and tapping techniques on the top layer of muscles in the direction of blood flow to the heart. They may also move your joints gently to improve range of motion. Whereas deep tissue massage, as the name suggests, is used to treat long-lasting muscle tension and the therapist applies slow strokes using intense pressure to reach deeper layers of the muscles.

Massage can be particularly therapeutic during menopause because, at a time when we feel out of kilter with our bodies, much like yoga, it can help restore a sense of connection with our physical selves. Moreover, because it uses touch, it reminds us that we deserve to be nurtured and cherished even as our bodies seem to be rebelling against us. Research shows that massage promotes better sleep and can reduce anxiety too. If you're using a therapist for the first time, it's wise to check if they are registered at **www.cnhc.org.uk**.

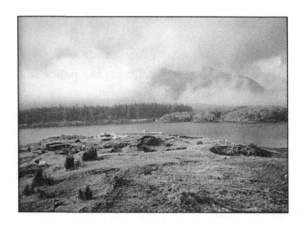

7.   'U' is for Upkeep

What risks do we need to be aware of in postmenopause, and what can we do to keep ourselves fit and well as we age?

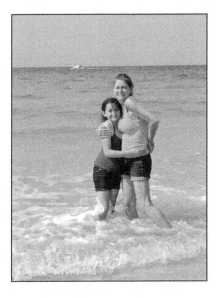

'The really frightening thing about middle age is that you know you'll grow out of it.' **Doris Day**

Once we've had twelve months without a period, we enter a different phase of our journey as women – postmenopause.   There can be problems associated with this time of life that cause us to worry – we are scheduled for regular mammograms and are advised to have our cholesterol levels, liver function and blood sugar checked, be aware of our BMI and continue with smear tests. If you read the wealth of literature out there it's easy to generate a very long list of symptoms and concerns, and possibly start to panic. **We're going to look at three of the most common issues – bone thinning (osteoporosis), raised blood pressure (hypertension) and weight gain – because we can do something about them.** (This is not to underestimate other symptoms, but given that postmenopause covers the years until – to call a spade a spade – we die, you'll appreciate the need to draw a line somewhere.)

It's very important to say however that for the majority of women, **postmenopause is a relief. Gradually hormones tend to settle and many women find they regain some sense of equilibrium after years of hiatus.** I'm now in postmenopause and would verify that life is a picnic for me these days compared to the perimenopause.

'Aim to relax and enjoy your postmenopause,' says Patrick. 'You've earned it! Let me thus keep the advice simple: **if you have an unexpected pain, bleeding or you find a lump anywhere in your body, then please see your doctor.** Otherwise, diet and exercise are the mainstays of a happier, healthier life post menopause, and this chapter provides a good overview moving forward.'

We'll also look at skin care – let's face it (oh dear, another pun), no book on ageing can avoid mention of wrinkles – and stress relief.

7.1 Osteoporosis

From the moment we are born, our bones are in a state of flux, breaking down old cells and building new ones. But the rate of turnover doesn't remain the same throughout our entire lives – bone density peaks at about the age of 30, then starts to slow.

As women approach menopause, our ovaries produce less and less oestrogen. And the less oestrogen we produce, the more our bone cells break down, which raises the risk of osteoporosis, or bone thinning, and also of bone fractures.

Osteoporosis has become more common as life expectancy has increased. Around 40% of women will suffer an osteoporotic fracture during their lifetime.

Can osteoporosis be prevented?

'Prevention is better than cure', so the saying goes, and we don't have to take this news lying down. Just the opposite, in fact: we need to get up, get moving and start making plans for keeping our bones as strong as possible. Apart from the menopause and natural ageing, there are a number of factors that may increase bone loss and bone thinning, including heavy smoking, excess alcohol intake, low body weight and a family history of osteoporosis. Whilst we may not be able to alter our family history, there's a lot we can do to help care for ourselves otherwise. It's a familiar story – **cutting back on alcohol, being careful to maintain a healthy body weight and stopping smoking can all make a big difference, as can diet and exercise.**

Q&A

Sarah: How is osteoporosis diagnosed?

Patrick: Osteoporosis tends not to be noticed until a fracture occurs, most commonly at the wrist, spine or hip. Ordinary X-rays of the hip and spine may suggest that the bones are thin but are not accurate enough to diagnose osteoporosis. The best test is a bone density (DEXA) scan. This is simple and painless.

Treating osteoporosis

If you are diagnosed with osteoporosis, as with so many effects of menopause, the first thing to look at is your lifestyle. Does it need to alter? If, after doing so as best you can, your risk of fracture *still* remains high, there are several effective pharmaceutical options which can reduce your risk by as much as 50% if started within five years of menopause. Some types of medication may be better for you based on your health history than others, and there are differences in the dosing schedules and method given, so you're advised to discuss the options with your doctor.

TIP: Once we've broken one bone we're at greater risk of breaking another, so cut your chance of falling in the first place. Clear your home of clutter so you're not tripping over shoes and boots left in the hallway or wires running between your desk and the door. Fix the lighting so you can see your way at night. If a lightbulb needs changing or you have to reach into a high cupboard, don't perch precariously on furniture hoping for the best. Make sure you have a stepladder that it is secure and that someone else is in the house, if possible, in case you do have an accident.

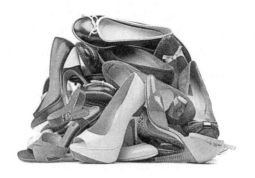

7.2 High blood pressure

It's important to understand whilst menopause transition is completely natural, it has a significant impact on the body. One reason is that oestrogen helps protect women from high blood pressure (also referred to as 'hypertension'). Once we stop menstruating and oestrogen falls, so blood pressure tends to rise, sometimes steeply.

At this point you might be thinking: *so what*? If my blood pressure is a bit high, why is that a big deal?
High blood pressure doesn't have obvious physical symptoms like hot flushes or aching joints, so it doesn't bother me.

Truth is, when women reach 45, we hit a statistical marker. It's probably one you weren't aware of: it's when our risk of stroke and heart attack begins to climb. Hypertension makes us more susceptible to both, and this is why high blood pressure can be cause for concern. **As we move into the menopause years, oestrogen is no longer protecting us the way it once did,** yet most women don't even *think* about the possibility of heart attack or stroke until they're much older – by which time, to put it bluntly, it may be too late.

The intervening years are when we can benefit enormously from being vigilant. Get your blood pressure checked regularly at your doctor's surgery, and if it proves unhealthily high, you'll need to bring it down.

TIP: Some people suffer from 'white coat syndrome' and get anxious about having their blood pressure taken by a doctor, which can lead to false readings. Monitoring your blood pressure in the comfort of your own home can help.

Blood pressure monitors are widely available for personal use (and are not too expensive), so if you're concerned, it may well be worthwhile purchasing one.

Tackling high blood pressure

Aside from medication, which your doctor would have to prescribe, there are four ways we can help lower blood pressure ourselves:

- We can lose weight
- We can take more care about what we eat and drink
- We can do more exercise
- We can reduce stress

Notice how these tactics overlap? Not only can we reduce our risk of osteoporosis in a similar way, **by making these changes we're likely to have an impact on conditions we've only space to mention in passing: diabetes, rheumatism and arthritis.** Even our chances of developing dementia and certain cancers will lessen.

So let's move on to the first of these, and see how we can tackle something that I, personally, have found a problem in postmenopause...

<u>**7.3 Weight gain**</u>

'Since the menopause I have gained two stone and I find this terribly upsetting. I was a size 8 until I was 40 and now I feel very fat. I find it hard to lose any weight.' **Annie, 50**

I'm in the same boat. Not that I was *ever* a size 8, but I have put on weight recently, and I can't seem to shift the extra pounds. Many of the women I spoke to in the course of writing this guide have said similar.

'One of the biggest shocks of the menopause was my body changing. From having a slim, quite boyish figure, I put on 10lbs. My body shape changed over a few months and I suddenly got breasts. I also put on weight on my middle, so I felt completely out of proportion. Eventually I decided something had to be

done, so I went into this little specialist lingerie shop and I said, 'I've put some weight on and for the first time in my life I think I need a bra,' and she said, 'Menopause?' and I said, 'Yes,' and she nodded and said, 'Mm. It happens a lot.' I was 47, and I didn't expect that. Looking back, getting a bra felt like the first step in accepting that my body was different.' **Holly, 54**

- Research indicates that depleted oestrogen may cause body fat to be redistributed, hence unexpected changes to our body shape.*
- Laboratory animals with lower oestrogen levels tend to eat more and be less physically active.
- Reduced oestrogen may lower metabolic rate so the body no longer creates energy as efficiently.
- Lack of oestrogen may also cause the body to use starches and blood sugar less effectively, which can increase fat storage and make it harder to lose weight.
- Sleep deprivation is common in menopausal years, and can lead to cravings for sugary/starchy foods.

We often compound this situation ourselves. Once we hit middle age, we're less likely to exercise. Some estimates indicate that around half of the physical decline associated with old age is due to lack of physical activity. We also lose muscle mass, which lowers our resting metabolism, making it easier to gain weight. This means that **to use the same energy as in the past and achieve weight loss, we have to *increase* the amount of time and intensity we're exercising**. For someone like me, who doesn't like exercise half as much as eating cake, this is bad news. Though at least it's not my mind playing tricks on me; it *is* harder to lose weight after the menopause.

7.4 Diet and exercise in postmenopause

At this point you could be forgiven for wincing, 'Ah-oh, here come the hardcore diet and exercise plans.'

Fear not. One look at the author photo opposite reveals that I'm no gym bunny, and I think it would be unfair to suggest you follow a regime I couldn't undertake personally. So, I'm *not* going to insist that

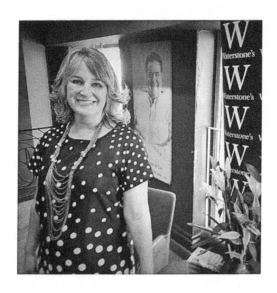

you start rising at the crack of dawn to go running, nor that you stick to a rigid diet. I'm inclined to think a 'little bit of what you fancy' doesn't cause much harm and put that theory into practice perhaps rather too often. Given I'm not likely to be entering the Olympics anytime soon (and neither, come to that, is Patrick), we'll keep our philosophy and tips for postmenopausal health simple.

Here's the philosophy

- Although this natural life transition can be uncomfortable, it in no way needs to herald the end of your vim and vigour.
- Often your level of energy and sense of wellbeing will be dictated by your lifestyle choices and attitude.
- In the context of the menopause, general health and fitness go a long way in reducing symptoms, which is why we've mentioned them repeatedly in this book.

Moreover, making time to look after yourself isn't anything to feel *guilty* about. Keeping your body and mind healthy is not *that* different to making sure your car is serviced or your computer is backed-up. I'd even go so far as to say that keeping yourself well is as much part of being a responsible, self-sufficient adult as other pursuits we often value more highly such as working hard or looking after others.

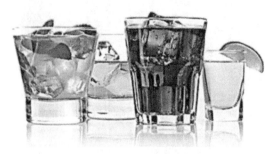

So how does this manifest itself in terms of what to eat?

Here's the advice on diet

- **Minimise alcohol consumption.** Alcohol can lower your body's ability to absorb calcium and can raise blood pressure, so if you drink, keep it to a glass a day.
- **Cut back on caffeine.** If you want to prevent osteoporosis and reduce hypertension, drink less coffee, tea and caffeinated soft drinks. (You should avoid high-caffeine energy drinks entirely.) Caffeine causes your body to excrete calcium more quickly and speeds up your heart rate which increases blood pressure.
- **Reduce salt.** Like caffeine and alcohol, salty foods can cause you to lose calcium and speed bone loss, as well as intensifying hypertension. Processed and canned foods tend to be high in salt, so limit your intake. When you do eat these foods, look for low- or no-salt-added brands.
- **A good calcium intake** is important at all ages; for women after the menopause the basic daily requirement is roughly the equivalent of a pint of milk – any sort. You also need **a good supply of vitamin D** to help absorb calcium. You can get vitamin D from just a few minutes of sunlight and from fish, oysters, and packaged foods that have been fortified, such as cereal. If you're not getting enough calcium or vitamin D from your diet, you might like to consider supplements.

- Increase your intake of foods that contain **naturally occurring phytoestrogens**, such as whole grains and beans. These may provide some symptom relief for postmenopausal symptoms by acting as a weak form of oestrogen in your body. Also aim to include soy, oats, wheat, brown rice, tofu, almonds, cashews and fresh fruits and vegetables.

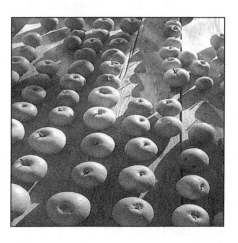

Don't

- **Succumb to diet/binge cycles** – this will cause great highs and lows in blood sugar and is likely to increase mood swings, irritability and anger.
- **Eat excessive sugar** as it limits your liver's ability to metabolize oestrogen and impairs the immune system – avoiding processed foods is a good way to reduce your intake of sugar.
- **Eat excessive commercially-raised beef, pork and chicken** because these meats contain a high amount of saturated fats and decrease the body's ability to metabolize oestrogen.

TIP: 'Don't allow the fact it's supposed to be harder to shift weight put you off trying. I felt so dispirited hearing that I didn't bother trying to lose anything and for a long time was heavier than I was happy with, believing there was no point dieting. Eventually I thought I'd give it a go, and I came up with my own variation on a Mediterranean-style of diet which was similar to my usual diet but healthier and with fewer calories, and I was surprised to find that it wasn't so hard after all. I've lost a stone and a half over four months, so it is possible, and I feel much better. I'd like to encourage other postmenopausal women in that respect.' **Lucy, 60**

If all this still sounds too complicated and you prefer your advice in even more of a nutshell (another pun, pray forgive me), **make sure you have a varied, balanced diet, eat regular meals, cut down on alcohol and caffeine, and drink more water**. Or, if all else fails:

'My best fashion advice to older women? Have a good haircut. It makes such a difference to how you look and feel.   **Sheila Hancock**

Here's the advice on exercise

'Other than stopping smoking, no matter what age we are, exercise is probably *the* most important thing anyone can do to improve overall health and wellbeing,' says Patrick. 'Just make sure to work within your own limits, which maybe running a marathon or having a gentle swim, whatever you're able to do.'

Physical activity reduces cognitive decline and improves mortality, helps prevent and reduce bone loss, and plays a key role in reducing your risk of many types of cancer. Exercise can also prevent your heart from stiffening as you age and thus reduce the risk of heart disease. So, if you're not yet exercising regularly, now's the time to start. Physical activity:

- Burns off stress hormones such as adrenaline
- Tires your muscles, reducing excess energy and tension
- Forces healthier breathing
- Releases endorphins which are natural antidepressants and improve overall mood
- Reduces feelings of tension, frustration and anger
- Improves the immune system
- Provides a healthy distraction from your worries
- Helps you get a better night's sleep and overcome insomnia

132

Studies show that exercise helps reduce feelings of stress, anxiety and depression in postmenopause while helping you avoid middle-age weight gain as well.

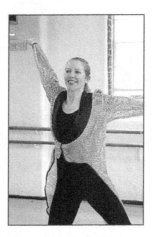

If you're naturally sporty (or, as above, dance-trained), then don't feel obligated to limit your ambitions because you're 50. 'There's no doubt that a brisk 30-minute daily walk and regular yoga sessions are hugely beneficial to women's health,' writes Ronnie Hayton in *The Guardian*. As a passionate club runner, she feels a bit depressed that the exercise recommended in menopause is often so very gentle. 'It is inconceivable to me, having turned 52, to consider that during the vigorous and vital years leading up to the cessation of menstrual periods, women should be any less sporty than before. We need to focus on the fact that our bodies are as strong and capable as ever and that we are not going to let ourselves be beaten by sometimes feeling a little hot as our ovaries readjust.'

Good advice, though I'd reason that activities like yoga don't *have* to be gentle and easy – I've a yoga teacher who demonstrates fearsome flexibility and stamina – and some women experience more than 'sometimes feeling a little hot' at this time of our lives. If you're up all night with night sweats, you could be forgiven for not putting an eight-mile run top of your agenda the next day.

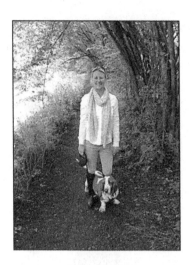

I would also add that 'exercise' doesn't have to mean sports. Anything that requires you to be active over an extended period of time can benefit your mental and physical health – so gardening, going for a walk with the dog and doing DIY or housework all count if you go about them with gusto.

- **The British Menopause Society advises regular weight-bearing exercise** to minimise risk of osteoporosis, e.g. walking, skipping or sports such as tennis or jogging. You'll get the most benefit if you vary your activities, which will make exercising more interesting, too.
- **Reduced mobility and poor balance increase the risk of breaking a bone**. Keeping fit and flexible is vital, and practices such as tai chi and yoga can help.

If you don't currently do much exercise, please start slowly and sensibly. A little light jogging or brisk walking can make a big difference to your mood and fitness levels; spraining an ankle will have the reverse effect. **Aim to build up so you do at least 20-40 minutes three or four times a week**.

Many women are self-conscious when exercising, so try not to worry about what you look like.

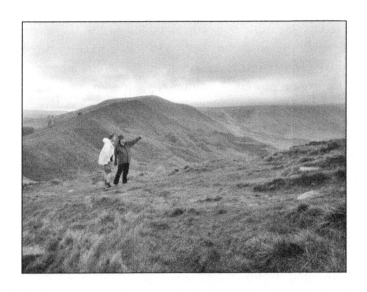

'I have opted out of continuing my salsa classes as they involved dancing with different partners, and I'm very self-conscious that hot flushes have the potential of turning me into a soggy mess when they take a hold of me! I do other forms of exercise instead and particularly enjoy cycling, as it offers a lovely cooling breeze as I whizz along.' **Chloe, 48**

Above all, **it's important that you *enjoy* whatever physical activity you're doing**. If that's cycling, not salsa, who is anyone else to judge?

7.5 Love the ageing skin you're in

When our skin becomes a little less elastic and our body shape starts changing, it creates a sense of ageing that we can't escape from. And because our society values supple skin, youth, beauty and fitness – particularly in women – the pressure to keep looking young can seem unrelenting.

'Sometimes it seems we'd rather look like we've come from outer space than appear old – there is so much negativity in our culture about ageing. Women lie about their age not just with words but with Botox and fillers because there's so much shame and fear about growing older.' **Juliet, 53**

The beauty industry is worth 16 billion in the UK alone, and skincare is the biggest sector with 30% of market share. We're bombarded by advertisements for anti-ageing products, many of which claim almost magical powers thanks to scientific-sounding ingredients, but how many of these actually work? Whilst there's certainly not space to sort all skin-care facts from fiction here, we can provide a few pointers. But first, let's clarify what's occurring biologically.

What actually happens to skin in menopause?

- 'Declining levels of oestrogen play a major part in skin ageing before, during and after menopause,' says clinical nutritionist and skin therapist Jane Atherton on **www.womenshealthadvice.co.uk**. It is 'responsible for collagen proliferation, production of natural oils in the sebaceous glands, skin cell turnover and controlling melanin, the pigment which gives skin colour.'
- She explains that within five years of menopause collagen drops by as much as 30%, leading to lower skin density. The result is often visible lines and a loss of firmness or sagging.
- In addition, falling oil production can cause dryness, lower melanin control can increase age spots and a reduced cell turnover can make the complexion appear pale and dull.
- Women often experience flushing during menopause, which can lead to redness and broken capillaries. Rosacea, caused by irregular hormone levels, is treatable.
- Stress can cause skin to become drier.
- Frustratingly, at the same time all this can be going on, some menopausal women find their skin is much more reactive than it used to be, which makes it harder to find products that are right for them.

Here's what you can do about it

But before you dial up the nearest plastic surgeon or bulk book the Botox, the good news is that not every woman experiences that much change in the texture and appearance of their skin. Moreover, **the lifestyle changes already mooted in this chapter can help offset some of these issues**.

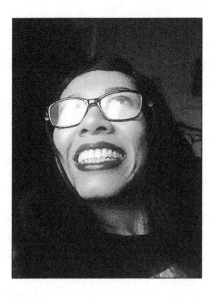

In addition you might like to consider the following:

- Nutritionist Jo Lewin says that nuts such as almonds and seeds such as pumpkin and sunflower contain nutrients such as vitamin E, zinc and calcium, along with oils, which may help prevent dry skin.
- Omega 3-rich foods such as salmon, sardines, flaxseed and walnuts contain essential fatty acids which support healthy cell membranes to hold water.
- Greek yogurt has nearly twice as much protein as regular yoghurt, and protein helps keep skin firm.
- Broccoli and other fruit and vegetables high in vitamin C help to stimulate collagen production.
- Vitamin E is an antioxidant that helps protect skin from damage by free radicals. Avocado, nuts and vegetable oil are all good sources of vitamin E.

- Exercise will boost circulation, and yoga or meditation can counter the stress which contributes to dry skin.
- Limit salt and sugar which adversely affect collagen, and dehydrating coffee and alcohol.

Product-wise, the terminology can be baffling and the choice overwhelming. We haven't space to explore all the options, but here are a few simple skin-care suggestions.

- Many personal care products contain not just fragrance but sulfates, propylene glycol and triclosan, writes beauty industry expert Dara Kennedy in *Huffington Post*. She recommends that if you're finding your skin is more sensitive than it used to be, you avoid these ingredients.
- Many products contain peptides which are 'endocrine disruptors' – put plainly, this means they interfere with our hormones. In menopause we've enough of that going on already, so again they're best avoided, particularly with regard to body moisturizer. Coconut oil is a good, widely available alternative.
- Retinol is an animal form of vitamin A, and is often used in products which aim to treat fine lines and loss of firmness, and research shows it is effective at conditioning and moisturizing.
- If your skin is sensitive and dry, retinol products may not be the best solution. A good alternative would be an oil-based serum that's naturally rich in vitamin A (a simple tip is to look for rose hip oil on the ingredient list).

Also, it's important to remember that the menopause is *not* singularly responsible for ageing our skin. (Look at men!) Skin ageing is influenced by several factors including genetics, environmental exposure, smoking, hormonal changes and metabolic processes. All factors together act on the alterations of skin structure, function, and appearance. Of these, research shows UV radiation is the single major factor in skin ageing.

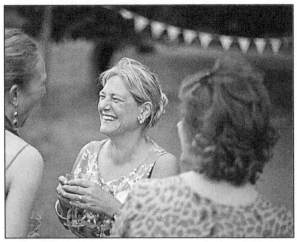

Photograph John Knight

TIP: Slap on the sunscreen: dry skin, wrinkles, moles and skin cancers can all result from too much sun, so keep skin healthy with sunblock of SPF30 or higher. Remember some healthy sun exposure is important to produce vitamin D, but if you think an overcast day means you don't need sunscreen, think again. Skin-damaging ultraviolet light can penetrate clouds, fog, even snow.

Alternatively, you might like to heed my octogenarian mother's advice. When I asked what she thought was the secret of her own relatively smooth skin, she said, 'Darling, there are no wrinkles on a balloon.' I view this as justification for ensuring my own face remains nice and plump and from time to time saying, 'Ooh, go on then. Pass the cake.'

7.6 Stress relief

We've already mentioned that in our middle years we're often pulled in different directions by the demands of work and family, and this can be especially hard if we feel we don't have the physical and mental resources we once did.

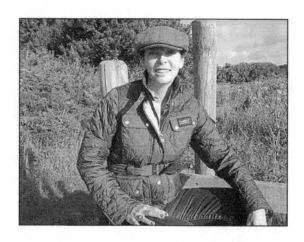

Emotional stress can wreak havoc on your hormonal balance at any stage of your life, while also making symptoms like insomnia, anxiety and depression worse. Any strategy that helps you reduce stress is a good one, and if you're someone who suffers a *lot* from stress, again, you might find *Making Friends with Anxiety* (both the book and the group) helpful.

'Buy yourself some candles, the biggest, softest blanket in the world. Have baths every day, use essential oils. Allow yourself the time and space to become familiar with the woman you now are.' **Holly, 54**

- **Each day, try to relax with a stress-reduction technique.** Exercise, yoga and acupuncture, along with deep breathing, guided imagery, meditation or even relaxing with a good book can all help regroup from stress. There are many tried-and-tested ways, so experiment and see what works best for you.
- **'A problem shared is a problem halved'**, so the saying goes. Stress can cloud our judgement and prevent us from seeing things clearly, **talking things through with a friend, work colleague or even a trained professional can help us to find solutions** to our problems and put them into perspective.
- **Writing can be a great way to take control.** Note down what's worrying you and come up with as many possible solutions as

you can. Decide on the good and bad points of each then select the best solution.

- At times we can feel overburdened by our 'To Do' list and this is a common cause of stress. Accept that you cannot do everything at once and **make a list of all the things that you need to do and list them in order of genuine priority**. Note what tasks you need to do personally and what can be delegated to others. Record which tasks need to be done immediately, in the next week, in the next month or when time allows. By editing what might have started out as an overwhelming and unmanageable list, you can break it down into a series of smaller, more manageable tasks spread out over a longer time frame. Hopefully you can remove some chores completely. **Delegate tasks or dump them.**

- A common cause of stress is having too much to do and too little time in which to do it. Despite this, how often do you find yourself agreeing to take on additional responsibility? I know I do. **Learning to say 'no' to additional or less important requests can go a long way to helping reduce stress.** It can be hard initially, but practise makes perfect.

- **Rest if you are ill.** If you are feeling unwell, do not feel that you have to carry on regardless. A short spell of taking it easy will enable the body to recover faster.

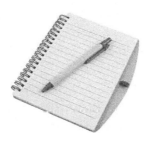

8.   'S' is for Sexuality

Whether you are alone or with a partner, good sex – however we define it – can enhance health and self-esteem. But what if intercourse is painful or you just don't fancy it anymore?

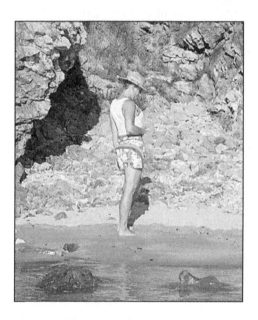

About a third of women lose interest in sex during the perimenopause, and around 40% lose interest in sex during the menopause itself. Yet sexual energy is part of what makes us human, and for most women is closely bound up with our sense of identity and attractiveness, so this shift in desire can have a big impact on how we feel about ourselves.

Although loss of libido is very common, many of us feel embarrassed to talk about it with our partners and peers. The same is true of vaginal dryness. Figures vary – according to www.patient.co.uk it's estimated that four-to five years after the menopause, up to 50% of women experience symptoms due to 'atrophic vaginitis' (a distinctly unappealing term if ever I heard one, given to 'atrophy' means to waste away and decline). This often makes it painful to have sex. According to a survey by Menopause Matters the numbers are higher –

they found that as many as 88% of menopausal women have a problem with vaginal dryness, and that 80% of respondents who were sexually active had been led to avoid sex for this reason. In either case, it's a *lot* of women. However, only around one in four of women with these symptoms actually seek medical help.

These are the 'secret symptoms' of the menopause, and we might learn to live with them because it makes our toes curl when we think of visiting the doctor about them, but shying from talking doesn't mean they go away. Quite the opposite: keeping schtum can compound negative feelings such as shame, guilt and self-loathing, which can make us feel less sexual still. So even if the topic makes you squirm, please don't stop reading. If we can't discuss these subjects in a book about the menopause which can be read in privacy, we'll find it hard to be open anywhere else, and there is help out there if you want it.

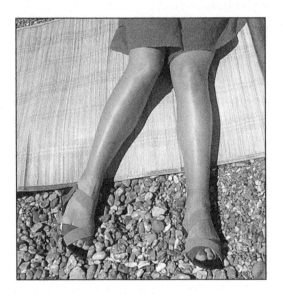

8.1 Loss of libido

'I'm not sure that being post-menopausal has changed my view of myself in terms of being a woman no longer able to bear children as I only ever wanted the two we have, and my husband had a vasectomy a year after our son was born, but I no longer view myself as a sexual person.' **Stella, 58**

Female libido is complicated. What makes any one of us desire sex varies so much I could spend the rest my life writing about it. (Which might be fun, I guess.) But even if I were only to focus on myself, I'd have my work cut out: what makes me feel sexy varies day to day, according to what I've eaten and drunk, who I'm with, what I'm wearing, how happy I am, if people have been nice about my books (or horrid), what's going on with my family and friends, how warm or chilly the weather is, if I've a writing deadline, if I'm on holiday and so on. I don't feel the same about sex now, at 53, as I did at 42. Neither do I feel the same about sex today as I did yesterday. My sex drive fluctuates, and always has. I expect you're similar. So **if ever there was an area of the menopause where 'one size does NOT fit all' in terms of solutions, it's when our libido is the issue**. All we can hope to do here is explain *why* our sex drive is often affected by the menopause and offer some pointers, just as we've done for every symptom we've covered thus far.

Why does our libido drop as a result of menopause?

- **Before menopause, in theory our sex drive peaks just before and after ovulation.** (It makes sense in terms of ensuring the survival of the human race.) When our periods stop, oestrogen dips, and those 'revved-up' days in our cycle are gone.
- **Less oestrogen also means less blood flow to the vagina, which causes a reduction in its elasticity and function**. Your vagina changes in shape, becoming shorter and often narrower, and you might lose some pubic hair. The walls of the vagina get thinner and lubrication decreases, resulting in dryness, higher risk of irritation, reduced resistance to urinary and vaginal infections and painful intercourse. And if it hurts to have sex, is it surprising that we don't want to?
- It's not just oestrogen that drops – **progesterone is also integral to maintaining sexual health**. When levels become low during menopause, the resulting irregular periods, fatigue and other menopause symptoms can cause loss of libido.

144

- **Our sex drive is also partly governed by testosterone**, which might surprise you, as it did me, because it's a hormone we tend to associate with men. However, women produce testosterone too; it's mostly produced in the ovaries and adrenal glands and plays a crucial role in our libido and overall experience of sexual pleasure. It contributes to our sense of wellbeing and energy levels; it can improve mood and outlook and increase feelings of confidence and assertiveness. When testosterone levels fall in tandem with oestrogen and progesterone, the overall result is that we may well respond less to touch and find it harder to get aroused. There is emerging use of testosterone for treating female loss of libido, but it is an unlicensed indication which your GP may be reluctant to prescribe. However a consultant might.

- **This can be compounded by other menopausal symptoms** such as night sweats, hot flushes, insomnia, mood swings, depression and anxiety. Dr Dawn Harper, presenter of Channel 4's **Embarrassing Bodies**, says that if we are waking up drenched in sweat several times a night and are chronically sleep deprived, then that is a good reason for wanting to get to sleep the moment our heads hit the pillow.

- **The physical changes that happen with ageing often don't help**. Dry skin, greying hair, middle-age spread – all these can lead to a poor body image and erode self-esteem.

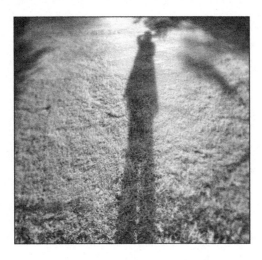

'I guess I'm "lucky" in that my skin and hair remain good, but I certainly know that weight gain around the midriff means I feel less attractive and sexy.' **Juliet, 53**

'I feel invisible and dowdy even though I take good care of my appearance. I lack confidence, but this is only since the menopause.' **Annie, 50**

- Then there's the rest of our lives: **a woman's interest in sex is affected by a multitude of factors** including stresses at work, concerns about money, worrying about what the kids are up to – you can fill in your own circumstances here.
- **Being in a long-term relationship can contribute too**. The 'Empty Nest Syndrome' can be a boost to romance but equally easily bring relationship problems as we turn the spotlight back on our relationship in a way we may not have done for a couple of decades. There are exceptions, but rare is the couple who feel as driven to have sex as often after twenty or thirty years together as they once did.
- **Medications** such as antidepressants and high blood pressure treatment can impact libido, as can ongoing health conditions like diabetes and heart disease…

…and so it goes on. Before we know it, we've amassed quite some list. I don't know how you felt upon reading it, but writing it made me feel it's a miracle that *any* of us women going through the menopause ever want sex at all!

According to the following US survey, only half of women of 50-59 have had intercourse in the last year, so if you've not been feeling the urge, it indicates you're far from alone.

Age	*50-59*	*60-69*	*70-79*	*80+*
Masturbated in previous year	54%	46%	36%	20%
Had intercourse (penis–vagina) in previous year	51%	42%	27%	8%
Received oral sex in previous year	34%	25%	9%	4%

*In a 2009 national survey of 5,045 older adults published in *Journal of Sexual Medicine* (2010;7[suppl 5]:315-329).

'I don't have any desire, need or urge to have sex. I find myself looking for close affection; for hugs, cuddles, holding hands etc. Thankfully my husband seems to feel the same and although we rarely have actual intercourse we are intimate with each other. We have discussed our lack of intercourse but are both agreed that it's OK. In discussions with friends my age it appears that most of them have no urge any more either, so I don't feel we're that unusual. Whilst I envy couples my age who still have an active sex life, overall I am happy that my hubby and I remain so affectionate.' **Stella, 58**

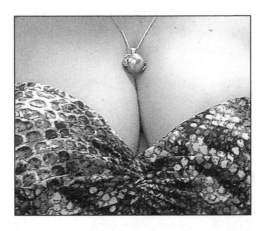

'I don't like my whole self – I need to lose weight – but I do like bits of myself in isolation, so I can see I'm still sexy.' **Diane, 44**

Let me take this opportunity to say that some women feel no difference in their libido to speak of, and continue their sex lives as before. Nonetheless, in western societies sexuality is often considered the domain of the young, and the idea of older women having and enjoying sex can sit uncomfortably with some of us. In Victorian times women tended to be portrayed as passive sexually (Queen Victoria is rumoured to have told her daughter to 'lie back and think of England') and sex was deemed solely to be for reproductive purposes.

Since the work of Kinsey and other sexuality researchers in the late 1940s perceptions of older people's sexuality have changed, but it still seems more acceptable for older men than older women to be sexual. According to Clinical Psychologist Eike Adams, the menopause is often described as a very negative time, especially in medical literature. On the other hand, feminists and women-centred writers celebrate the menopause and subsequent years as a time of positive change, without the commitment to childrearing, offering the chance to find new fulfilment. He points out that the experience for each individual woman is likely to be somewhere in the middle, believing that most of us continue in older age with what we used to like doing when we were younger. Hence if you enjoyed having sex it is most likely you will continue, but if you didn't, you might be relieved to stop. I disagree with the last assumption, as the experience of having sex might be very different for some of us if it becomes painful. What was once enjoyable could well no longer be so.

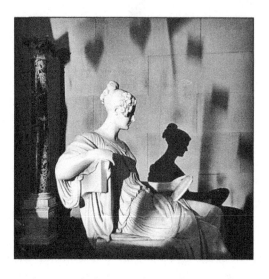

'After suffering whatever the menopause threw at me without much help and no complaint, nothing could have prepared me for the shock and misery that vaginal atrophy has caused me – post menopause. I had read nothing of any substance on this subject. All you hear people harping on about is hot flushes and mood swings. So after a year of being in absolute agony and four misdiagnoses later, I get diagnosed with it and guess what? There's **still** very little information out there about it. Also, treatment is very difficult – because I have a womb! I'm hearing four differing opinions from gynecologists and GPs. I don't know what to do and it's very traumatic. Damn right women need to talk more and so do the medical profession. We need to be prepared for this shit!' **Maggie, 54**

'Being asked to contribute to this book has given me the courage to mention thus unmentionable too. After a painful and upsetting smear test last year - which shook me - I asked my GP and after an exam she commented that it was "rather dry up there". I was 51, slim-ish and fit: I teach dance. This development was a shock. My husband takes meds for depression/anxiety which hasn't done anything for our sex life, leaving me feeling less of a woman and this diminishment of my womanliness has hit really hard. I knew it could happen, but not so "young". I don't have children and feel neutralized and embarrassed and no, there's not much out there to advise or support us with this difficult and intimate aspect. Add Fluoxetine to the mix and self-pleasure wasn't a success, even after Poldark! I no longer take that, but I wonder what life will be like on the other side and fear it's more of the same and worse.'
Bernadette, 52

Q&A

Sarah: What if we don't want sex – does it matter?

Patrick: Decreased interest in sex may be temporary or long-term, and here it's beneficial not to beat yourself up about something that is so common. For some women, there's a total lack of interest, even revulsion to sex. But if you don't feel like having sex, getting caught up in feelings of guilt or remorse or nostalgia is not going to make your desire any greater. It's more likely to create a cycle of negative thinking and then it will become a self-fulfilling prophecy. If you can be open to the possibility of change and transformation, keep talking to your partner and gently trying new things, you may well find your libido returns. It may be you're both fine with less penetrative sex, preferring alternative ways of expressing your love and affection and that's fine too. But if you'd like to resume an active sex life, treatment can be helpful. I'd strongly recommend talking to your GP or practice nurse about the options. I've helped patients with this issue and it's given them a boost to be able to take pleasure in physical contact with their partners again.

Of course not every postmenopausal woman is in a relationship, or heterosexual, and the truth is there is no age limit for sex, either alone or with someone else. Just because we're not part of a couple doesn't mean we don't want to enjoy pleasure – we may still want to masturbate. So, before we decide to throw in the towel and join a nunnery (to mix a metaphor or two), let's see what treatments might help us to be more sexually active.

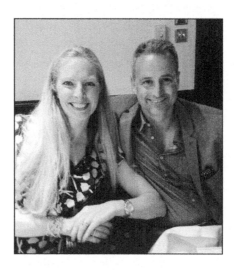

Remedies

Often a few modifications in diet and exercise will not only help alleviate loss of libido, but corresponding stress and anxiety as well. Yet Channel 4's Dr Harper points out it often takes more than that. 'Sex is meant to be fun! Why would you want to have sex if it's jolly well uncomfortable?' She feels it's important that we continue to experience pleasure.

Blogger Angie MacDonald agrees, and describes how she had to do something about her low libido or risk losing her relationship. After a long battle she was referred to a consultant and prescribed bio-identical HRT including testosterone, and a month later her depression had lifted and libido returned. For Angie, taking one small action to do something to improve her libido helped her reclaim her sexuality and lust for life and she's keen that other women follow her example.

If you find the idea of starting a conversation with your doctor about these intimate issues embarrassing, you might like to write out a list of symptoms and take it with you. There is a good one you might like to download and print out on **www.menopausematters.co.uk**.

Gynaecologist Edward Morris, chair of the British Menopause Society, says simple treatments can change lives.

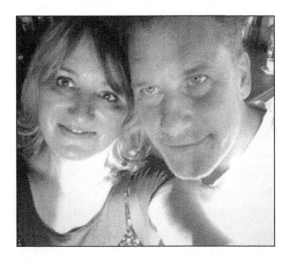

He believes that because the root of the problem for women going through the menopause is a drop in hormone levels, and that the best way to treat this problem is often to go directly to the hormonal source.

- **Traditional HRT** can ease hot flushes and other symptoms that leave you feeling not so sexy, but it doesn't seem to rekindle desire for most women.
- **Topical HRT** includes vaginal oestrogen creams or tiny oestrogen tablets that stick to the vaginal walls and deliver a more reliable dose. While both contain enough oestrogen to restore the vagina to its former condition and reduce the risk of infections, a year's cumulative dosage of the tablets is only the equivalent of one tablet of HRT. Women can use them for as long as they choose. Surprisingly, a new locally acting oral agent is said to be available soon.
- **Over-the-counter products** such as vaginal moisturizers and sexual lubricants can also help hugely. There are many different kinds of lubricant on the market these days and so you can shop

around to find one that works for you. If you find you experience irritation with one product, try a plant-based lubricant with as little scent as possible. There's a good guide to lubricants here.

TIP: If you're embarrassed purchasing lubricant over the counter, this is where internet shopping comes into its own. Why not look around online? www.lovehoney.co.uk is woman-friendly, as are www.sh-womenstore.com and www.annsummers.com. Packages are discretely wrapped so you don't need to worry about postal delivery. Even Sainsbury's sells lube!

- **Avoid potential irritants** such as perfumed soaps, bath products and vaginal deodorants. This will help stop sex from being painful, which can help a lot. Nonetheless...

- **...take the focus off intercourse**. If you don't already, spend more time on foreplay. Expand your repertoire. Try massage and oral sex.

- **Masturbation isn't just a crutch to use in place of sex with a partner. It is a self-affirming sexual activity** and is eminently useful in helping to discover different routes to sexual pleasure. Being more playful with your vagina and clitoris (maybe stimulating them with fingers first), can increase the vaginal fluids and make the vagina wetter. And as you may well already know, **vibrators aren't just for penetrative sex**, so you might find one designed for clitoral stimulation does the trick for you.

TIP: Again, this is where online shopping is a sex-lifesaver! Some sites have customer reviews of their products to help you decide which products might work well.

- **Also, treat your body kindly, making time for self-care and relaxation** (which we looked at in Chapter 7). Don't believe that only a slim starlet can be sexy. The photos of women in this book (all of whom are 45 and over) prove otherwise, don't you agree?

'As a feminist, I find the idea that only youthful women can be desirable and desiring frustrating – we seem particularly hooked on this idea in the west, where middle-aged women are encouraged to spend thousands of pounds and go through painful surgery in the attempt to stave off signs of ageing. As for the notion of "growing old gracefully" – if that means dressing in a twinset and pearls – pah! I intend to remain disgraceful as long as I feel like it and the body is willing.' **Juliet, 53**

• **Get talking** – and not just to your doctor. Chatting to your peers can make a massive difference – my bet is you'll be amazed how many have gone through something similar, and you'll feel less weird and alone. If you're as open with your friends as I am with a few of mine, you might even be able to share some tips. **I'm a firm believer that women can have a positive effect on one another.** No matter if we're gay or straight, single or in a couple, we can illuminate and enlighten, get involved in joint physical activities, share   discoveries about healthy diet for menopause and involve others in our social circles in healthy lifestyle changes. **To my mind, this is what 'Making Friends with the Menopause' is all about.**

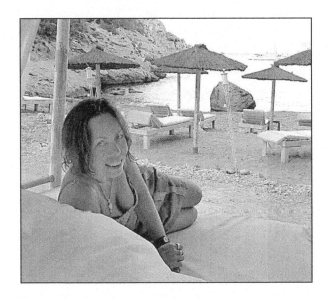

- It's also important to **communicate with your partner**. If you feel awkward about it, it might help if you ask him to read the last section of this chapter, which has been written with men in mind.

'Laughing about sex is really important, and sharing with friends. Being able to turn up at a mate's house and say, "I'm raging like a bull at my partner, there's no way that I'm up for anything today," or "Right now, I'm horny as hell!"' **Holly, 54**

- If these strategies aren't sufficient, **you might consider seeing a sex therapist**. Your therapist can help you sort through feelings about sex and ageing, issues with a partner, or medical conditions that impact on sex, and she or he can suggest additional ways to help you feel sexual. To find a psychosexual councillor in your area go to **www.counselling-directory.org.uk**.

8.2 Lesbian women and the menopause

Lesbians and heterosexual women certainly have the same problems in menopause – hot flushes, mood swings, vaginal dryness, the lot – but lesbians who are in a relationship may find it easier to negotiate solutions in terms of their sex lives because their partners can have similar issues. On the other hand, that they're going through the menopause together might make it trickier.

'You think one menopausal woman in the house is tough? Try having two! Joking aside, when we're both moody it can be dire, but having a partner who ***really*** *understands what I'm going through is good in some ways. Luckily we've both suffered, because I imagine if one of us had breezed through the whole experience, the other could have felt pretty resentful. We're friends with another gay couple with a seven-year age gap, and I think they might be a lot worse off because they're going to go through it twice. I imagine that'll put quite a strain on their relationship.'* **Carol, 50**

The important thing to remember is that even though you might both be going through menopause, you won't be experiencing it the same. One of you may have hot flashes and irritability, the other brain fogginess and heart palpitations, says *Lesbian Life* contributor Kathy Belge. Again, there is no 'one-size-fits-all'. Of course there are lesbians who stay vital through menopause, just as with straight women. They don't have the negative feeling that their sexual life is over and take a more holistic approach to this period of change in their life.

Nonetheless, stress is known to have a negative effect the symptoms of menopause, so a woman who has to deal with homophobia might have a harder time than a straight woman without that factor, sex educator Dr Carol Queen points out. Thus the experience of a lesbian from a conservative area, dealing with homophobia on a daily basis, is likely to be very different to someone from a gay-friendly place (such as Brighton, where I live) who goes out dancing every week.

If your GP doesn't seem very gay-friendly, you're perfectly entitled to change your doctor (**www.healthwithpride.nhs.uk** has good information on your rights in this respect). It's possible for doctors to achieve awards for their equality work and many have gay-friendly noticeboards, so if you're unhappy, switch.

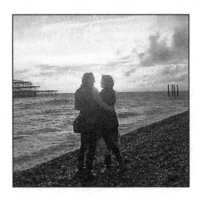

8.3 Men and the menopause – a section for male partners

'Any man who can see through a woman is missing a lot.' **Groucho Marks**

There are some men who think the menopause is women's business and there's no need to be informed or involved in it. Sorry, but that's rubbish, and if you're a bloke reading this, I hope (for your partner's sake, should you have one, if nothing else) you're not that insensitive. If hitherto you've done an ostrich because you're embarrassed by it all – which many women (see introduction) can be inclined to as well – now's the chance to shake the sand from your feathers and face the situation together. Women's insecurities are often linked to the reaction of their partners so it'll probably be better for both of you.

When it comes to sex, once her periods have stopped, a woman may experience dryness and intercourse can become painful. Partly as a result, she might not feel like having penetrative sex. This can lead to her not feeling very good about herself and worried about how it may affect her relationship with you. The menopause can be a time when a lot shifts for a woman, both physically and psychologically. She may also think: 'I'm struggling to understand myself, how on earth can I expect him to understand me?'

'Having erratic periods has not been the worst thing about the menopause. The worst thing has been not recognising myself physically, mentally, emotionally – having to buy new clothes and change my wardrobe at a time when I didn't know who I was – I hadn't realized how much my identity had been connected to the way I looked. I had been stylish... and to suddenly find myself with a very mature woman's body was a huge shock.' **Holly, 54**

One of the key ways that you could show you care is to point out the things you've noticed that have changed and genuinely concern you. Psychosexual therapist Denise Knowles says that she became incredibly clumsy and her husband noticed, and said: '"Are you alright? It's not like you". Just the relief that he'd noticed was good.' So let her know you're not being disparaging and that it's something you'd like to be looking at and working through together.

'My husband buys lube for us to use. We found a good one with no perfume that doesn't irritate me, but I find it a bit embarrassing as it's only available from a sex shop in town. So he gets it. I like being taken care of in this way – it shows a gentle understanding. Or maybe he just likes an excuse to visit the shop!' **Juliet, 53**

If you've not really talked about your sex life lately, it may feel awkward at first. Knowles suggests you ask one another how you are feeling. For example, 'I get the sense you don't want to have sex with me as much these days, and I wondered how you feel about it?' Then listen to what she says. If she's upset, give her space to think and come back to the discussion another time.

Also, trust me (as a postmenopausal woman I've experience of the mindset) just because your partner doesn't feel as much like having intercourse, it doesn't mean her desire to be *with you* has dwindled. For many men sex is reassuring, so it can be hard to understand this.

There's more to sex than penetration

'If I ask people what makes a satisfying sex life, they usually say it's about penetrative sex and orgasms,' explains Denise Knowles. 'But this isn't necessarily what sex and intimacy is all about.' So – if you don't do this already – you may have to find new ways of exploring sex and learn how to be intimate without penetrative intercourse once your partner has been through the menopause. **Some couples kiss a lot, going back to how things were before their sexual relationship and relearning ways of displaying intimacy and affection. Others might like oral sex or using a vibrator to turn them on.** We women need to feel we're still desirable and that you still want to get close to us.

One reason your wife or partner has not been to the doctor may be because she's scared or being an ostrich too. So why not offer to go to the GP with her? Even if they can't help at the surgery, the GP may refer her to the local menopause clinic, which generally has doctors, specialist nurses and counsellors on hand to tackle problems. In any event, it'll show you care, and that you're on this road together.

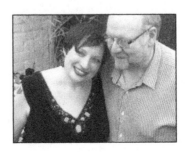

9.   'E' is for Emergence

We're nearing the end of our journey together, dear readers. But before we go, let's look at the entire lived, felt experience of the menopause, and see what significance it might have for us in terms of life as a whole.

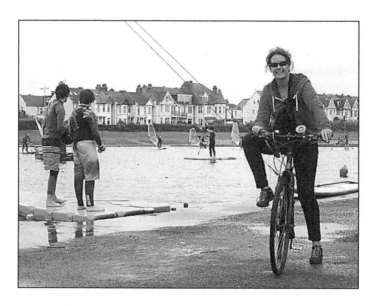

*'It's interesting to compare myself with other menopausal friends, as I feel a bit better now. More like I know who I am again. When my symptoms were at their worst, the fear for me was, "Oh my god I'm going to feel this crap for the rest of my life" and I'd like to reassure other women that they won't. I don't feel the same as I did before. I feel larger – I **am** larger – but I don't feel as sad, or as swamped by a sense that I've lost something.'* **Juliet, 53**

'Every single part of my life has altered. My body, my wardrobe, my work, my relationships... For years I felt I wasn't in control of anything – until now.' **Holly, 54**

9.1 Acting our age

Rules about age are changing. As Marianne Williamson says in her book, **The Age of Miracles: Embracing the New Midlife,** while a growing segment of our population is living to be over 100, it's not that our lives are getting extended at the end, but *in the middle*.

Consider the statistics: in 1900 Britain, life expectancy for women at birth was 50, 100 years later it was 81. Whilst a much higher infant mortality rate in the past accounts for some of this difference, it's nonetheless the case that women are living much longer, and this is a trend that continues; those aged 20 now are three times more likely to live to 100 then those who are now 80. This means that the menopause is taking place increasingly centrally in terms of a woman's lifespan. 100 years ago it came close to the end of life, for my mother (born in 1933) it came 2/3 of the way through. For our daughters, if trends continue (and

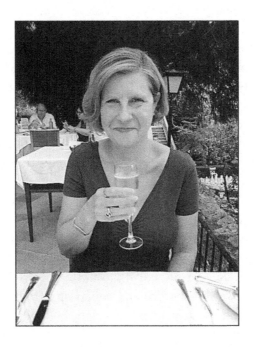

there's no global disaster to alter this picture), it will happen in the middle. An ageing population creates problems, true, but modern medicine, a better understanding of diet and exercise and cosmetics also allow us to stay healthier and look better longer. As Williamson says, this creates a new space in which to create what it means to be 'you' in the middle years of your life. And these middle years are when,

I'd venture to suggest, we *do* have a choice. We can spend our middle years looking back ruefully at our youth. We can spend thousands of pounds or dollars on procedures – going under the knife to restore the pertness of our breasts, injecting poison to recreate smooth skin, but ultimately this just obscures the truth.

Mariella Frostrup wrote recently about ageing in *The Guardian* newspaper, observing that the unhappiest of her generation often seem those most afraid to evolve away from the fashions and ambitions of their earlier years. She feels that the greatest obstacle to equilibrium is our reticence to change, encouraged by a society that regards clinging on to the raft of youth as the only way to stay afloat.

We can't stop evolution doing what evolution does, says author and psychotherapist Susan Brayne, because at a certain point in a woman's life her body ceases to be fertile, resulting in a massive drop in oestrogen levels which affects every part of her body, including her brain. Brayne points out that no matter how much Botox, or what face-lifts and HRT she might use to try and beat it, a woman will age. The problem is that we live in an anti-ageing, youth-obsessed culture, where it's all about what we look like and what we have, rather than who we are. Brayne believes that as a society 'we have lost respect for the whole human experience, which includes ageing.'

Frostrup feels that since she turned 50 it's as if she is living in two separate worlds, a tangible one filled with energetic, sexy, adventurous, hard-working and active friends and a wider society where neither she nor her contemporaries seem to exist at all. And she's certainly not the first to observe that older women often feel invisible.

Given this state of affairs, it's easy to see why those whose identity and self-worth is particularly bound up with their appearance fight to look young. Each woman has a right to do this if she chooses, yet let's not deceive ourselves: it's a battle we're destined to lose.

'It annoys me when people say "Even if you're old, you can be young at heart!" Hiding inside this well-meaning phrase is a deep cultural assumption that old is bad and young is good. What's wrong with being old at heart, I'd like to know? Wouldn't you like to be loved by people whose hearts have practised loving for a long time?' says

Susan Ichi Su Moon in **This is Getting Old: Zen thoughts on Aging with Humor and Dignity.**

Perhaps it's helpful to see life as circular in this regard. I know logic says life is linear, but bear with me. If we see life as a line, then it's easy to chop off certain sections of it, cut them apart from one another, like a ribbon snipped by scissors. Over there we've childhood, aged 0-16, then youth, 17-40, then middle age, or whatever. Menopausal women are thus sundered from our younger sisters, left looking at that piece of ribbon, that separate entity, with dismay.

But if we see life like a circle, as Paula Gunn Allen suggests in her essay in *Red Moon Passage,* then all of life has a space and relationship within that circle. She explains that menopausal women have a place within that great hoop of being and relationships to everything else within it. Thus we don't leave the circle when we go through menopause; nor is there one circle for women aged 15 to 39 and another for women over 40. If life is seen this way, the thinking that says passing through the menopause somehow puts one outside the realm of a constructive or purposeful life is contrary to the natural order of things.

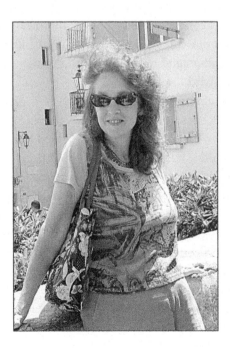

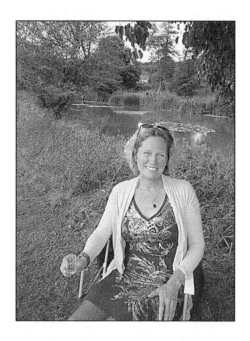

'You only have one life, but if you do it right, once is enough.' **Mae West**

Menopause is a major landmark of ageing, says alternative health practitioner, Ray Peat. He feels that if its meaning is radically misunderstood, then a coherent understanding of ageing is unlikely, and without an understanding of the loss of functions with age, we won't really understand life.

Whether we choose to see menopause as a great tragedy or a transition into a deeper way of living is up to us, writes Carol S. Pearson in *Red Moon Passage*. The choice of which it is depends largely on what which we *think* it is, because both could be true.

What these wise women and men have to say is spot-on: **to deny ageing – of which the menopause is a perfectly natural part – is fruitless**. Much of the fear around menopause is connected to fear of our own mortality – that we're no longer able to give life is a stark reminder that we are going to die.

'In every parting there is an image of death.'
        George Eliot, extract from **Scenes of Clerical Life**

Men don't have such a brutal wake-up call in this regard as their fertility declines more gradually, but we do. So instead of resenting and berating men for seeming to have a different mindset in middle age to our own, perhaps it's better – more empowering – for us to embrace our wisdom. After all, it means we're more able to appreciate the transient nature of being. And, as we briefly touched on when talking of mindfulness in Chapter 5, we can waste a lot of energy trying to recapture the past or worrying about the future.

The important time to focus on, surely, is *now*. If we're going to make it to 80 or 90 or 100, it strikes me as a huge waste to spend our 50s, 60s, 70s or whatever wishing we were 20, 30 or 40, or nervous and agitated about what is going to happen. We have a choice in this regard; we don't have to put our focus and attention there, and I hope reading this little book has helped open your eyes to this possibility in the same way that writing it has helped to open mine.

9.2 Postmenopausal zest

The American Anthropologist Margaret Mead called it 'menopausal zest' – the rush of energy, both physical and psychological, that some women feel after menopause. 'There is no greater power in the world than the zest of a postmenopausal woman,' she said.

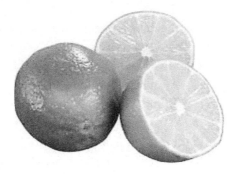

Journalist Barney Beardsley writes eloquently in the *Daily Mail* about how being postmenopausal meant her body felt her own again, after being on loan for years to the weird processes of puberty, pregnancy and menopause.

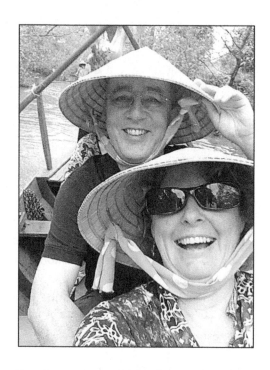

She describes how the sudden, drastic dip in oestrogen which comes at mid-life felt like withdrawal from a powerful drug and that five years of cold turkey was no picnic. She had a dry mouth and dry eyes, a suddenly accelerated heartbeat, a body temperature flushing high then swooping low, and at that point couldn't imagine how things would change again, that the dark tunnel of mid-life would open into a landscape of infinite and new possibilities. Now she is 55, however, she is experiencing an unfamiliar and somewhat unexpected profound sense of wellbeing. Yet she's under no illusions: she says she has the body of a 55-year-old, with all the creases, sags, bumps and crinkles that entails. But it is also a contented body, with curves again, and there is a sense of strength returning, a kind of sly and sensual delight in being who she is. Her sleep is better, her appetite lusty, she has a spring in her step.

This renewed vigour makes postmenopause a natural time for us to take stock of our lives. It's important to take advantage of this wake-up call; that we pause, consider and listen to ourselves.

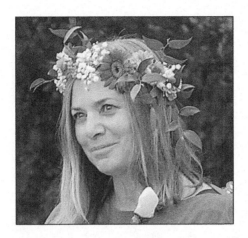

'Women may be the one group that grows more radical with age.'

Gloria Steinem

In *Sex, Meaning and the Menopause,* Susan Brayne[i] describes how she got together a group of women to talk about this time of their lives and that it became clear menopause was anything but a purely negative experience. Some said they felt liberated and excited; others more creative and self-accepting and several saw it as the chance to revisit hopes and dreams, to reassess what mattered to them. '"It's okay to be me," said one. "I like being selfish in a positive sense," said another. A third said she was enjoying moving out of the role of mother, and becoming more of a mentor. "I like spending more time out in the world as who I *am*, rather than who I am expected to be."'

You might like to take a fresh look at your relationships, your work, the way you're caring for your own health and using your time. Ask yourself:

- Is the way I am spending my time meaningful to me?
- Am I using my physical energy well?
- Am I intellectually stimulated as much as I'd like?
- Is there anything I wish to learn or study?
- Are my friends people whose company I actively enjoy?
- Are my partner and I in tune at this time of our lives?
- Are there places I want to travel?

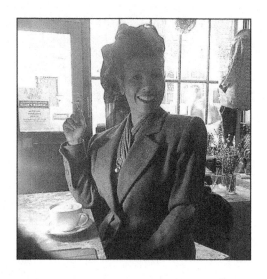

I don't suggest you do this in a rush, or to formulate a list of grievances. Instead, try to think about these issues in a non-judgmental way. If you hear your inner critic sniping 'yes, there are places I want to travel, but my partner would never go with me', that's only going to create resentment and a sense of disempowerment. Step back, if you can. It takes time to work out what you want, so allow yourself to ponder as you go about some gentle activity or as you're drifting off to sleep. Consider ways around obstacles. Let your imagination flow. And at the same time as you explore your own needs, be open to compromises. As Professor Randy Pausch said before he died (aged 47), 'It's not the things we do in life that we regret on our death bed, it is the things we do not...We don't beat the reaper by living longer but by living well, and living fully – for the reaper will come for all of us. The question is: what do we do between the time we're born and the time he shows up?'

And remember, we may feel imbued with 'postmenopausal zest', but still we tire more easily as we age, so we have to let go of being all things to all people. Get clear about what you most like doing.

'Lately, I've been doing a different kind of creative work. My writing is more nurturing of other people and I'm more interested in building a community so in that regard I'm less go-getting.' **Juliet, 53**

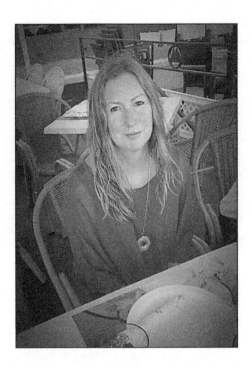

'The great question that has never been answered, and which I have not yet been able to answer, despite my thirty years of research into the feminine soul, is "What does a woman want?"' **Sigmund Freud**

9.3 A wiser woman

If we see menopause as a purely bodily event, then it's easy to get caught up in the symptoms and the sense of loss. Yes, there are upsides physically to coming out the other side – after our periods stop (a relief in itself for many), fibroids shrink, PMS disappears, menstrual migraines cease and so on. There's no doubt that compared to perimenopause, postmenopause is a *much* less rough hormonal ride. Nonetheless, if we focus solely on the physical aspects of menopause, we're likely to end up hooked by the fact that we're no longer young or able to give birth. Brayne says that too much emphasis is put on physical symptoms rather than psychological issues, and she's got a very valid point.

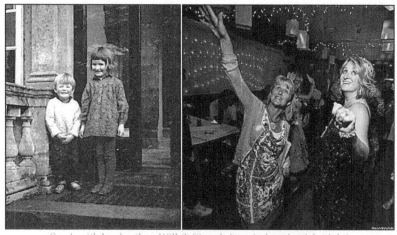

Sarah with her brother, Will (left) and sister-in-law Annick (right)
Right image by John Knight

'The great thing about getting older is that you don't lose all the other ages you've been.' **Madeleine L'Engle**

If, however, we see menopause as bigger than that, as a time of psychological and spiritual transformation, then it's much easier to reframe it as a positive -- or, more accurately, multifaceted -- experience. Most of what women today have to read about menopause sits firmly within a western scientific and medical tradition, writes Brayne, which might be termed as a masculine, logical approach. The danger with this, she feels, is it has all but banished the softer, more nebulous feminine qualities of sensitivity, intuition and creativity.

This book aims to balance both. At times, yes, we've been logical -- personally, I don't see rationality as unhelpful -- but we've also given space to consider emotional responses and an alternative point of view. Surely there's room in our lives for both, and both are valid? Yin and yang, masculine and feminine, call them what you will.

'Each woman's experience of the menopause is both individual and similar. It is a bit like having a vast list of things that might or might not happen and it's almost impossible to predict. I feel the menopause is not shared or talked about enough as a celebration and rite of passage -- which, given that half the world's population will go through it, is astonishing. It's a HUGE transformation --

168

physically, emotionally and psychologically – and, as this book so eloquently puts it, the key is to be friends with the changes rather than to fight them. Apart from anything else, that's macho language, not feminine, and one of the most important things during this phase in a woman's life is self-care. Nurturing not battling, understanding and working with the body and the mind, not using the language of being at war with our own amazing, life-giving bodies. ' **Julie, 55**

Above all, I believe that it's *awareness* that matters. As Paula Gunn Allen observes in *Red Moon Passage*, in order to make a successful passage through menopause, women need to be aware of what is happening to them. Just as a young girl might be frightened if she doesn't understand why there is blood between her legs, an older woman may be scared if she doesn't understand the menopausal phenomenon.

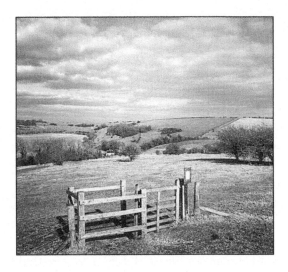

'There's no right or wrong way to make this journey. It's about finding your own route through the menopause and however that is, it being OK.' **Holly, 54**

In this book Patrick and I have endeavoured to take some of the fear away. Knowledge is power, and I hope as we near the last page, you agree.

9.4 Join the conversation

'Never doubt that a small group of thoughtful, committed citizens can change the world. Indeed, it is the only thing that ever has.'
Margaret Mead

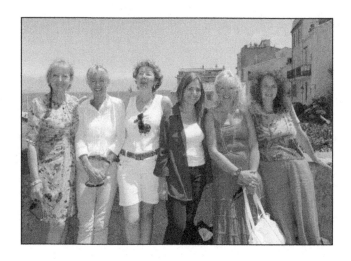

Time and again throughout this book we've seen how the menopause is not a dysfunction but a natural life change. Talking – and often joking – with other women about the menopausal and postmenopausal symptoms you're experiencing can lighten the load and increase understanding, and hearing from others who've been through it can provide reassurance that you're not alone. I hope that's part of what this book, ***Making Friends with the Menopause***, with its interjections and insights from other women throughout, has given you.

Last but by no means least, I'd like to say thank you for reading. I hope this little book has helped unravel a complicated subject, and to given you pointers for where to seek further help. If so, I would appreciate it if you could **leave a review on Amazon.** This will help others find it and it's useful to hear what readers thought. I also suggest **you keep this book close to hand**, so if you're having a bad day you can reach for it.

Finally, a reminder of that **Facebook group** I've mentioned so repeatedly. *Making Friends with the Menopause* **is at www.facebook.com/groups/makingfriendswiththemenopause/** and is the place to go to share tips and seek advice from other women going through the transition too. You can also join my mailing list at www.sarah-rayner.com and be the first to hear about author events and book offers.

In the meantime, Patrick and I would like to end by wishing you health and happiness.

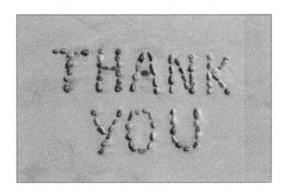

Acknowledgements

First and foremost, I'd like to thank Patrick for all his help with this book. It's been a pleasure to work together and I look forward to future collaborations. A big thank you to Leigh Forbes, Laura Wilkinson and Zoe Woodward for their help with editing and layout, my mother, Mary Rayner, for her help with proof reading. My friends who read this in draft get a mention too – Nicola Lowit and Karen Palmer as does Tom Bicât, my husband.

I'd also like to thank all the women featured. There are those whose individual stories and anecdotes pepper this guide and those who let me use their photographs. I couldn't have done this book without you. Personally, I feel if anyone doubts that women can blossom through menopause and beyond, they only have to look at the pictures of the women in this book to be convinced that yes, they can.

About the authors

Sarah Rayner

Sarah Rayner is the author of five novels including the international bestseller, *One Moment, One Morning* and the two follow-ups, *The Two Week Wait* and *Another Night, Another Day*. She is currently working on her sixth novel.

Friendship is a theme common to Sarah's fiction and connects her non-fiction titles too. In 2014 she published *Making Friends with Anxiety, a warm, supportive little book to help ease worry and panic*. This was followed by *Making Friends with the Menopause* and *Making Peace with Depression* with Kate Harrison and Dr Patrick Fitzgerald. In 2017 Sarah set up the small press **www.creativepumpkinpublishing.com** and the imprint now publishes the *Making Friends* series.

Sarah lives in Brighton with her chef husband, Tom. You can hook up with her on Facebook, on Twitter and via her author website, **www.sarah-rayner.com**, where you can sign up for her mailing list to receive her *Making Friends* magazine with a free short story and mood-boosting guide.

Dr Patrick Fitzgerald
MB.BS MRCGP Diploma in Palliative Medicine

Patrick studied medicine in London and became a GP in 2007. He has a special interest in cancer and palliative care and has worked as a GP educator for Macmillan Cancer Care, in hospices and with community and hospital palliative care teams.

He is an advocate of patient-centred care, focusing on shared decision-making with patients. He feels the role of the GP is as medical translator and advisor, communicator, and, mostly, listener. He knows no more than the average GP about the menopause, so please do ask your GP for support if you have troublesome symptoms. If your GP can't help you, they will probably know a gynaecologist who can.

Useful websites

The menopause:
www.menopausematters.co.uk
www.marilynglenville.com/womens-health-issues/menopause
www.34-menopause-symptoms.com
www.empowher.com
http://menopausehealthmatters.com/
http://www.theperimenopauseblog.com/symptoms-of-perimenopause/

General health:
www.bupa.co.uk
www.childline.org.uk
www.netdoctor.co.uk
www.nhs.uk
www.patient.co.uk

Counselling:
www.britishpsychotherapyfoundation.org.uk
www.counselling-directory.org.uk

Sexual health:
www.sexualadviceassociation.co.uk

Sarah's websites:
www.sarah-rayner.com
www.creativepumpkinpublishing.com

Recommended reading

The Menopause:
Red Moon Passage: The Power and Wisdom of Menopause, Bonnie J. Horrigan
New Menopausal Years, The Wise Woman Way, Alternative Approaches for Women 30-90, Susun S. Weed
Sex, Meaning and the Menopause: a Book for Men and Women, Sue Brayne
The Stranger in the Mirror: A Memoir of Middle Age, Jane Shilling

Mental Health:
Shoot the Damn Dog, a Memoir of Depression, Sally Brampton
Depressive Illness, The curse of the strong, Dr Tim Cantopher
The Examined Life, how we lose and find ourselves, Stephen Grosz
The Unquiet Mind, a memoir of moods and madness, Kay Redfield Jamison
Sunbathing in the Rain, a cheerful book about depression, Gwyneth Lewis
Sane New World, Taming the Mind, Ruby Wax
The Mindful Way through Depression, Freeing Yourself from Chronic Unhappiness, Mark Williams, John Teasdale, Zindel Segal and Jon Kabat-Zinn

Additional articles of interest

The menopause:
http://www.theguardian.com/lifeandstyle/the-running-blog/2015/jan/15/all-change-running-fast-through-the-menopause

http://www.dailymail.co.uk/health/article-2956296/Menopause-lasts-14-years-Study-says-doctors-advise-women-symptoms-occur-longer-previously-thought.html

The perimenopause:
http://www.dailymail.co.uk/health/article-2324019/Menopause-The-unexpected-signs-youre-hit-it.html

Bio-Identical Hormones:
http://www.theguardian.com/books/2014/apr/11/jeanette-winterson-can-you-stop-the-menopause

http://www.fda.gov/ForConsumers/ConsumerUpdates/ucm049311.htm

Menopausal zest:
http://www.dailymail.co.uk/femail/article-2115112/Yes-menopause-hell-But-feel-sexier-ever.html

http://www.theguardian.com/lifeandstyle/2015/feb/22/mariella-frostrup-life-after-50

Men and the menopause:
http://www.dailymail.co.uk/femail/article-1292604/Yes-male-menopause-DOES-exist--time-women-took-seriously.html

On specific symptoms:

Anxiety:
http://www.telegraph.co.uk/health/wellbeing/11046587/How-to-detox-your-life-beat-anxiety-through-meditation.html

http://www.dailymail.co.uk/health/article-32984/How-treat-anxiety.html

Panic attacks:
http://www.dailymail.co.uk/health/article-2156928/How-control-panic-attacks.html

Insomnia/night sweats:
http://www.dailymail.co.uk/home/you/article-1324506/Why-change-isnt-good-rest.html
http://www.theguardian.com/lifeandstyle/2014/apr/19/tips-to-combat-insomnia

Depression:
http://www.nytimes.com/2014/08/16/opinion/depression-can-be-treated-but-it-takes-competence.html

http://www.huffingtonpost.co.uk/jamie-flexman/depression-mental-illness_b_3931629.html

References and sources

1. https://www.nice.org.uk/guidance/ng23/chapter/recommendations#managing-short-term-menopausal-symptoms
2. http://www.nice.org.uk/guidance/ng23/chapter/Recommendations#long-term-benefits-and-risks-of-hormone-replacement-therapy

The digital version of this paperback has links to source material throughout. If you've purchased this book through Amazon.com, you can download the ebook for FREE and access these links directly. If you are unable to do this and would like details of a source, please contact sarah.rayner1@btopenworld.com for a file with embedded links.

The 'Making Friends' series is available in paperback and digital format on Amazon worldwide. Several titles including this one and Making Friends with Anxiety are also available on audio via Audible and Amazon.

Making Friends with Anxiety: A warm, supportive little book to help ease worry and panic

'Simple, lucid advice on how to accept your anxiety' **Matt Haig, bestselling** author of *Reasons to Stay Alive.*

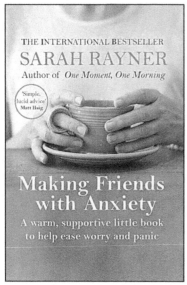

Drawing on her experience of **anxiety disorder and recovery**, Sarah Rayner explores this common and often distressing condition with candour and humour. She reveals **the seven elements that commonly contribute to anxiety** including adrenaline, negative thinking and fear of the future, and explains why it becomes such a problem for many of us. **Packed with tips and exercises** and offset by the author's photographs and anecdotes from her life, if you suffer from panic attacks, a debilitating disorder or just want to reduce the amount of time you spend worrying, *Making Friends with Anxiety* will give you a greater understanding of how your mind and body work together, helping restore confidence and control.

- Uses **Mindfulness-based Cognitive Therapy** techniques
- Includes **photographs** by the author to lift the spirit
- **Useful links** throughout, plus details of **helplines**
- Online support group with nearly 10,000 members

'Reads like chatting with an old friend; one with wit, wisdom and experience' **Laura Lockington, Brighton and Hove Independent**

Making Peace with Depression: A warm, supportive little book to lift low mood and ease despair

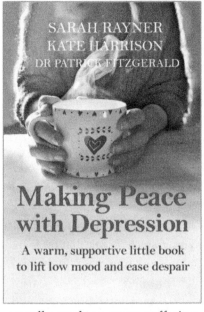

From the bestselling authors of *Making Friends with Anxiety* and *The 5/2 Diet Book* comes a clear and comforting book for sufferers of depression.

If you're experiencing very low mood, you can end up feeling very alone, desperately struggling to find a way through, but recovery *is* possible and friends Sarah Rayner and Kate Harrison, together with GP Dr Patrick Fitzgerald, show you how. They explain that hating or fighting the 'black dog' of depression can actually prolong your suffering, whereas 'making peace' with your darker emotions by compassionately accepting these feelings can restore health and happiness.

Sarah and Kate write with candour, compassion and humour because they've both been there and, together with Dr Patrick Fitzgerald, have produced a practical guide to support the journey to recovery. It explains:

* The different types of depressive illness
* Where to seek help and how to get a diagnosis
* The pros and cons of the most common medications
* The different kinds of therapy available
* Why depression can cause so many physical symptoms
* What to do if you suffer suicidal thoughts
* How to stop the spiral of negative thinking
* The link between poor self-esteem and depression
* And why hating depression can make it much worse

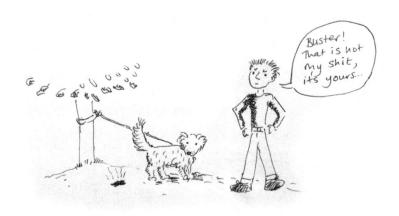

Fully illustrated by Sarah and reflecting the latest National Institute for Health and Care Excellence guidelines, *Making Peace with Depression* is much more than a memoir; it aims to help you see how low mood can feed on itself and show you ways to break that cycle by

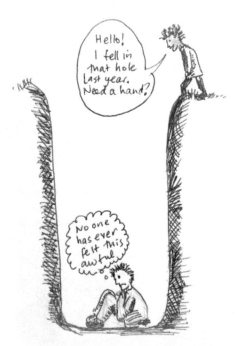

treating your body and mind with understanding and kindness. You'll find realistic suggestions on eating and exercise, advice on self-medicating with drink and drugs, as well as tips on reaching out and avoiding relapse, all delivered with a surprising lightness of touch. The result is book that doesn't shy away from the bleakness or difficulties of the subject but remains tender and life-affirming, offering hope and guidance through the darkest of times.

More Making Friends with Anxiety: Discover simple ways to occupy your hands and calm your mind

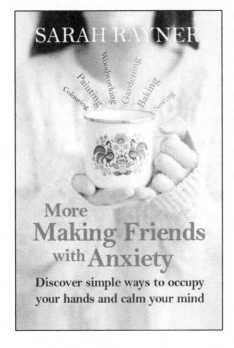

The follow-up to *Making Friends with Anxiety*, *More Making Friends with Anxiety* is packed with easy, practical things to make which will occupy your hands and calm your mind. Written with Sarah's trademark warmth and humour, *More Making Friends with Anxiety* will inspire and uplift you, nurturing mindfulness and positivity. And because each project can be completed in less than two hours, these activities are ideal for complete novices and children too.

* Paint Pebbles * Decorate glass * Make a Collage
* Sew a Simple Cover * Bake a Crumble * Carve Wood
* Plant a Windowbox * Make a Necklace * Look at Art
* Listen to Music … and more

Fully illustrated with photographs by the author and clear step-by-step instructions.

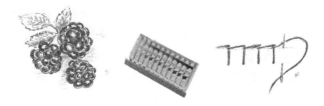

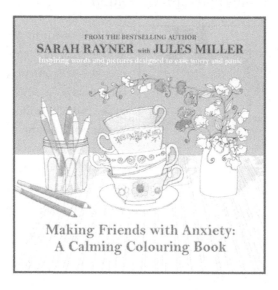

A beautiful adult colouring book packed with tips and insights to encourage mindfulness and ease worry and panic.

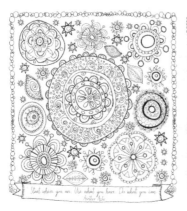
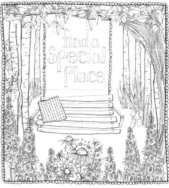

Making Friends with your Fertility: a clear and comforting guide to reproductive health

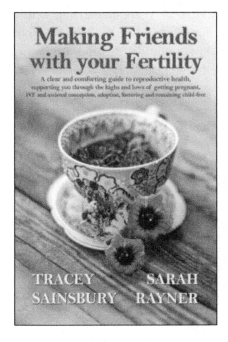

The onset of periods and puberty, egg and sperm production and preparing to conceive naturally, IVF and assisted conception – fertility counsellor Tracey Sainsbury and Sarah tackle them all with warmth and humour. Together they take you on a journey not just exploring what happens when things go well (through intercourse, orgasm and pregnancy), but also looking at situations where conception is not so straightforward, as it isn't for the 1 in 6 experiencing infertility.

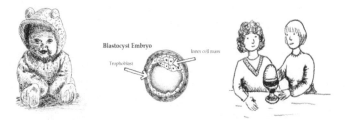

The result is a handy, practical primer, packed with tips, illustrations and real-life stories making complex issues less confusing and overwhelming, and supporting each individual so they can 'make friends' with their own fertility, in whatever form that takes.

'A brilliant and well-written piece of work.'
Francesca Steyn, Head of Nursing, The Centre for Reproductive and Genetic Health

Making Peace with Divorce: a warm, supportive guide to separating and starting anew

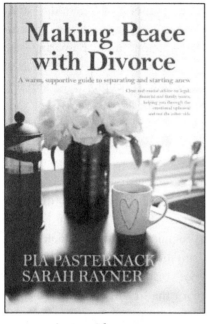

After 20 years of marriage, full-time mum Pia Pasternack came home one day to find a note on the doormat and her husband gone…

Heartbroken, this was the first of a series of revelations that left her and her children reeling. But gradually Pia built herself back up and together with Sarah Rayner, in this book Pia passes on the legal, financial and emotional lessons she learned. Together they guide you through sensitive issues such as whether to separate, how to break the news to children and how best to communicate with your ex.

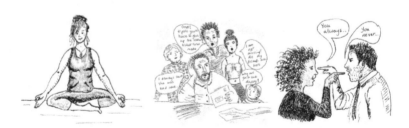

There is advice on finding a lawyer, filling in forms and reaching a settlement. Offset by Sarah's illustrations, the result is a guide that makes complex and distressing issues less confusing and overwhelming, so each individual can find peace with their own divorce or separation, thereby creating a happy and fulfilling future.

Making Peace with the End of Life: a clear and comforting guide to help you live well to the last

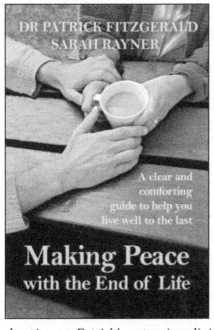

From GP and hospice doctor Patrick Fitzgerald and Sarah Rayner comes a book to support you and those caring for you in the last months, weeks and days of life. From the shock of diagnosis, through treatment options and symptom control to the process of dying itself, *Making Peace with the End of Life* tackles these sensitive issues with compassion and honesty. Full of practical advice and useful contact information, it will demystify how the NHS and Social Services work, so you can access the best support. And, drawing on Patrick's extensive clinical experience, it also looks at how communicating your wishes to those involved in your care can give a feeling of safety and control over whatever happens in the future.

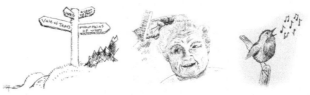

Offset by Sarah's illustrations and diagrams, the result is a clear and compassionate guide that makes complex and distressing issues less confusing and overwhelming, so each individual can live the life they have left with a greater sense of comfort and peace.

'Beautifully written – very gentle, personal and not at all frightening.'
Doreen O'Hara, COPD Specialist Nurse

International Bestselling Fiction by Sarah Rayner

One Moment, One Morning

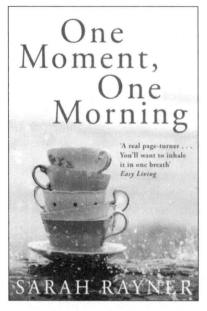

'Delicious, big hearted, utterly addictive, irresistible.'
Marie Claire

'A real page-turner... You'll want to inhale it in one breath.'
Easy Living

The Brighton to London line. The 07:44 train. Carriages packed with commuters. A woman applies her make-up. Another observes the people around her. A husband and wife share an affectionate gesture. Further along, a woman flicks through a glossy magazine. Then, abruptly, everything changes: a man has a heart attack, and can't be resuscitated; the train is stopped, an ambulance called. For three passengers on the 07:44, life will never be the same again...

'Oh, what a novel ! It will make you laugh and cry, it will make you want to call your dear ones to tell them how much you love them, it will make you buy it for all your friends. When you get to the end, Anna, Lou and Karen will feel like they are your soul sisters.' Tatiana de Rosnay, author of **Sarah's Key**

Available on Amazon worldwide and through all good bookshops

The Two Week Wait

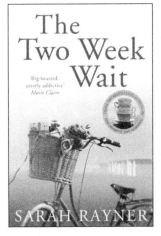

'*Carefully crafted and empathetic.*' **Sunday Times**

'*Explores an emotive subject with great sensitivity.*' **Sunday Express**

After a health scare, Brighton-based Lou learns that her time to have a baby is running out. She can't imagine a future without children, but her partner doesn't feel the same way. Meanwhile, up in Yorkshire, Cath is longing to start a family with her husband, Rich. No one would be happier to have a child than Rich, but Cath is infertile. Could these two women help each other out?

Another Night, Another Day

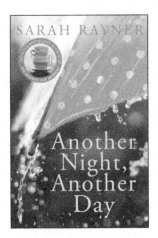

'*An irresistible novel about friendship, family and life's blows*' **Woman & Home**

Three people, each crying out for help. There's Karen, worried about her dying father; Abby, whose son has autism and needs constant care; and Michael, a family man on the verge of bankruptcy. As each sinks under the strain, they're brought together at Moreland's Clinic. Here, behind closed doors, they reveal their deepest secrets, confront and console one another and share plenty of laughs. But how will they cope when a new crisis strikes?

Made in the USA
Monee, IL
22 January 2021